CONTENTS

INTRODUCTION

Plant-Based Diet: there are so many things to know about the plant-based Diet, a real lifestyle that involves not only the choices at the table but also essential implications on what you decide. Here is a guide on how to make it your lifestyle.

Proper and balanced plant-based Diet: how to do it?

Find plant-based diet specialist or remote nutritional consultancy service created to satisfy the need and is aimed at everyone, with particular attention to pediatric patients, pregnant women and the elderly.

In any case, however, it is not necessary to consult a nutritionist simply for wanting to switch to a plant-based diet; it becomes so when you have specific needs. To stay healthy, on the other hand, it is essential to follow a varied and balanced diet.

Plant-based Diet and sport: is it possible (even at high levels)?

Not only is it possible, but even advisable. In recent years, more and more sporting, even at the highest levels, have chosen to exclude meat and animal products from their Diet, maintaining excellent results or even increasing them. To prove it, not only the numerous plant-based diet athletes at the Olympics but also the scientific evidence: be it amateur or professional - is not only advisable but even beneficial. For those who practice physical activity, a diet that guarantees energy is important necessary for training, but also integrating the mineral salts and vitamins that will inevitably be lost during physical exertion, as well as the fundamental proteins for muscle recovery.

Plant-based Diet and children NO danger to health

Many myths gravitate around the plant-based Diet, but the most widespread is that according to which it would be a difficult diet to follow, rigid and not suitable for children. Again, however, experts tell a different truth. The plant-based Diet is not only suitable for children, but it is also healthier compared to other types of diets. The most obvious benefits are mentioned by the American Academy of Pediatrics and concern the rarity of overweight and lower blood cholesterol levels in plant-based diet children. But in general, all international guidelines classify plant diets as healthy, even in children. However, if a child is fed an adequate and balanced plant-based diet, not only will he not face deficiencies, but will find numerous health benefits.

No danger even for plant-based Diet during pregnancy, on the contrary: this is a preferred choice, even for omnivorous women. This is because, as the expert explains, plant-based Diet is the one that exposes the fetus to fewer risks, such as endocrine disruptors or environmental pollutants. This, however, is not enough: the plant-based Diet is suitable for any age, even in the elderly. The advantages of this food choice in old age, among which the possibility to effectively prevent and treat chronic diseases such as diabetes, cardiovascular diseases, obesity and overweight stand out.

What do plant-based diet individuals eat?

Once you've discovered that plant-based Diet is advisable at every stage of life, it's time to find out what to bring to the table! First, it may be useful to draw up a plant-based diet shopping list, trying to understand how and with which foods plant-based diet individuals replace traditional ones. It is also important to check the labels, which often hide ingredients of animal origin hidden behind unclear alphanumeric abbreviations.

Understanding what plant-based diet individuals eat is quite simple, in reality: fruit, vegetables, oilseeds, and dried fruit form the basis of a 100% plant-based diet, to which foods can also be added (completely optional) like seitan, tofu, tempeh and the like. The plant-based Diet, therefore, is not only suitable for everyone and at any age, but it is also a collection of foods, flavors, and tastes that are often new and original, a must try!

Chapter 1: What is a Plant Based Diet?

In simple terms, a plant-based diet means consuming food that comes from plants. A plant-based diet does not include ingredients that come from animals, such as milk, meat, honey, or eggs. With a plant-based diet, it is now possible to meet your nutritional requirements with only natural and minimally processed items.

A plant-based diet includes fruits, vegetables, and tubers. A diet laden with veggies, fruits, tubers, and whole grains will help you diminish the harmful effects of many chronic diseases. For instance, did you know that a diet full of fresh fruits and veggies can lower blood pressure and control Type 2 diabetes?

You need not feel apprehensive about this change, because going for a plant-based diet does not necessarily mean that you will turn vegan. Neither do you have to give up on dairy or meat. It is rather an informed decision to primarily choose food items sourced from plants.

Plant-based diets like the Mediterranean diet have been proven to reduce the risk of certain cancers, metabolic disorders, and even heart disease. In older adults, a plant-based diet has also been effective in reducing the effects of depression and increasing physical and mental function.

How do You Start a Plant-Based Diet?

There are a few lifestyle changes one needs to do to start a plant-based diet. Going in too strongly will cause tension to build up only to be blown when a craving hits. Some may find it very difficult to follow but you only need to keep a few points in mind to achieve success.

Increase greens in your diet. A variety of vegetables are present for choosing to offer different flavors and textures for soothing your tongue. Pick vegetables regularly for meal bases and a replacement for unhealthy snacks. The crunchiness and flavors of some veggies might decrease the likelihood of eating junk food.

Most healthy diets don't just forbid the consumption of fats but instead tells you to replace bad fats which are derived from animals with good ones derived from plants. Seeds and olive oil are a good source of healthy fats which do not increase the body cholesterol levels.

Cut down meat, especially red meat as much as you can. You can still consume it if you are following a more lenient diet but it is discouraged. Replace your meat with seafood or tofu which can be a good substitute for it.

Rather than putting desserts on the table, you should place fruits or fruit dishes. They are a healthier option with the same hints of sugar to satisfy the sweet tooth. Some people crave sugar more, they can slowly cut off sugar from their diet by switching it for sweet fruits instead.

Replace everyday cow's milk for plant-derived milk such as soy, almond, rice or coconut. Milk is an important part of a diet that is impractical to fully remove from the diet.

Stay away from foods that have a lot of sugar like a Pepsi or are high in fat like french fries.

Also do not buy processed food because they are riddled with salt and sugar, which are enemies to your body.

Be aware that not every nutrient is being provided fully and arrange a replacement for that. Vit B12 is present in some cereal and in nutritional yeast. Iron is also less consumed so eat a healthy dose of cabbage, spinach or kidney beans to make up for it.

Nutrients in the Plant-Based Diet

Foods are made up of a mix of macronutrients (carbohydrates, fats, and proteins) and micronutrients (vitamins and minerals). The largest component of your daily intake should be carbohydrates. Fat makes up the next largest section, followed closely by protein. Since fats give you twice as much energy for the same volume, when looking at the portion size, fat and protein should be about equal.

Most people should aim for 60 to 70 percent carbohydrates, 20 to 30 percent fat, and 10 to 15 percent protein in their daily diet, with up to 20 percent protein for elite athletes. If your energy needs are about 1,500 calories, which I find to be the average of my clients, that works out to 225 to 263 grams of carbohydrates, 33 to 50 grams of fat, and 38 to 56 grams of protein per day. The specific percentage that works for you may be at the higher or lower end of those ranges, but the ranges are appropriate for about 98 percent of the population. Where you fall within the ranges may change a bit throughout your life and throughout the seasons of the year, so listen to your body. Despite some popular diet guides, there's most likely no benefit in going outside of these ranges. Even the biggest bodybuilders never need more than 20 percent protein, and it can in fact be harmful to your kidneys and general metabolism.

If you're like most people, though, you don't look at foods as carbohydrates or fats—but as rice or avocados. The cool thing about plant foods is that they're much more nutritionally balanced than animal foods, so it's easier to stay within the normal ranges listed earlier without having to meticulously track what you're eating. Let's look at the proportions of macronutrients in whole plant foods.

Carbohydrates

Some people worry about consuming too many carbohydrates by eating plant foods. Carbohydrates are your body's main source of energy and are completely healthy if you eat them in the form of whole foods (such as whole grains, vegetables, and fruit), since they contain lots of vitamins, minerals, antioxidants, water, and fiber. Fiber is also a carbohydrate, but its role is to facilitate digestion rather than give energy.

Whole grains and fruit have the highest levels of carbohydrates, with about 70 to 90 percent carbohydrate content. Eating a banana is an instant energy boost. The best food sources of fiber are psyllium or flaxseed and leafy green vegetables.

Protein

It's not nearly as hard as people think to get enough protein from plant foods. All whole plant foods have some protein in them. If you eat enough calories from a balanced and varied diet, and include legumes regularly, you should get more than enough protein and all the essential amino acids (which are the building blocks of protein). You do not have to combine different foods in a single meal to get the essential amino acids all together—a common misconception. If you eat different foods within 48 hours, the amino acids will get together to do their job.

Legumes, including beans, have the highest overall protein content of plant foods at about 18 to 25 percent; they are also important in plant-based diets because they provide enough of the amino acid lysine. Dark green leafy vegetables have a high proportion of protein at 40 percent, spices add tiny but important amounts of amino acids, and whole grains add a fair amount of protein to an overall balanced diet at 8 to 12 percent.

Fats

Your body needs enough dietary fat to function, maintain metabolism, and absorb and utilize minerals and certain vitamins. People with cold hands and feet, amenorrhea (missed menstrual periods), or dry skin, hair, or throat may need more fats in their diet, and particularly saturated fats like coconut oil. To be clear, eating healthy fat in reasonable amounts doesn't make you fat.

The best source of healthy fat is whole plant foods—avocados, nuts, and seeds (including nut and seed butters). These average about 80 percent fat. Whole grains and beans also have some healthy fat, and there are even small amounts in fruits, vegetables, spices, and pretty much every food. Oats, for example, are about 15 percent fat.

Oils are 100 percent fat and aren't something you necessarily need to eat, but they are great for carrying rich flavor and mouthfeel in a dish, particularly when you're transitioning to a healthier diet. If you use oils, it's best to keep them minimal and use unrefined oils like olive, coconut, sesame, and avocado. (Refined oils include canola, soy, sunflower, and corn oil.) You can easily sauté vegetables for two people with just a teaspoon of oil.

That doesn't mean you should never eat oils, though, and some people can actually benefit from concentrated fats. For example, flax oil or concentrated DHA might be necessary for someone with issues digesting and utilizing omega-3 fatty acids.

Chapter 2: Benefits of a Plant Based Diet?

A plant-based diet has proven health effects due to the composition of the foods. Reduced consumption of saturated fats prevents various diseases, including cardiovascular problems, high cholesterol levels, and obesity. The following are other guaranteed benefits of this diet:

Weight and BMI Control

Research studies conducted on the plant-based diet have revealed that people who follow it tend to have lower BMI or body mass index, reduced risk of obesity, and a lower chance of heart disease and diabetes. This is mainly because plant-based diets deliver more fibers, water, and carbohydrates in the body. This may keep the body's metabolism up and running properly while providing a good boost of continuous energy.

Back in 2018, a study was conducted on this diet plan and it was found to be the most effective for treating obesity. In that study, 75 people with obesity or weight problems were given a completely vegan plant-based diet and their results were compared with those consuming animal-based diets. After four months of this experiment, the plant-based diet group showed a significant decrease in their body weight (as much as 6.5 kilograms). They all effectively lost more the fat mass and showed an improvement in insulin sensitivity. Another study involving 60,000 individuals showed similar results with people on a vegan diet recording the lowest body mass index compared to vegetarians and animal-based dieters.

Lower risk of heart disease and other conditions

The American Heart Association recently conducted a study in which middle-aged adults who were on a plant-based diet were studied. All the subjects showed a decrease in their rate of heart disease. Based on the results of this research, the association has listed the following diseases which can be prevented through a plant-based diet:

Heart stroke

High blood pressure

High cholesterol levels

Certain cancers

Type II diabetes

Obesity

Diabetes

Plant-based diets also help manage diabetes as it improves insulin sensitivity and fights against insulin resistance. Out of all the 60,000 participants in the study, about 2.9 percent on the vegan diet had Type II diabetes, while 7.6 percent of participants following nonvegetarian diets presented with type II diabetes. From this observation, the researchers confirmed that a plant-based diet could help in the treatment of diabetes. It was also proposed that this diet can help diabetic patients lose weight, improve metabolic rates and decrease their need for medical treatments.

It was also suggested that doctors should recommend this diet as part of the treatment for people with type II diabetes or prediabetes. While medical treatments ensure short term results, the plant-based dietary approach offers long term results.

There's no need to count calories in this diet. It can be a tedious and time-wasting task that a busy person cannot afford. This diet simply allows some food and restricts the rest. A calorie doesn't tell much about the food, what nutrients are in it or is it healthy or not.

Plant-based foods are full of carbs and fiber which fills up the stomach quickly making you feel less hungry. You will consume less of the foods that will be no good for you like sodas or candies.

There is a higher quantity of water in plant-based food which increases body metabolism and reduces appetite. Water has many benefits, being hydrated makes you have better hair, skin and makes you look fresh.

By following this diet, you will not only help yourself in becoming better but also push the environment to progress in the right direction. A lot of pollutants come from Barnes and poultry farms. Making meat puts high stress on our planet and by consuming less of it, you are leaving less of a carbon footprint. Also by this diet, you are discouraging the use of meat as well.

It doesn't require any sort of investment and a person can begin it as soon as they decide to. Plant-based products are everywhere and even in a normal diet, take a big portion of it. Some dieting programs and fads take a lot of money from people giving only temporary results but this diet has shown to reduce the most amount of weight.

While there is no doubt that humans were meant to be eating fruits, vegetables and nuts from the beginning, a shift took place that introduced a large confusion, mixing humans with the omnivore species. Scientifically speaking, a plant-based diet is much more beneficial and less harmful for humans, which is why it is recommended to shift from meat to whole grains, legumes, vegetables and other nutritional foods of this kind.

Switching to a plant based diet is beneficial for many reasons. If you are suffering from any kind of illnesses or have obesity issues, you should focus on a plant based diet as a way to better your health and reduce your symptoms, if not cure the illness completely. Nutrition is a powerful tool that can be used for great purposes, such as helping relieve pain and health problems, improving metabolism and the immune system, as well as strengthen your body and improve your mood.

Even if you do not have any health-related problems, you should transition to a plant based diet as a means of preventive health building. The natural ingredients such as fruits, legumes or vegetables are full of nutritional values needed for the everyday functioning of our systems. In all cases, whole food is always better than processed food, as it does not contain any chemicals or unnatural substances that could be harmful to our health.

Besides boosting your health, a plant-based diet can decrease the risks of many diseases, among them the most serious ones such as heart diseases, type 2 diabetes and certain types of cancers.

Many studies at research facilities have proven these statements to be correct, such as, for example, a study conducted in JAMA Internal Medicine, which tracked over 70 000 people and their eating habits. This study has proven that a plant-based diet can significantly improve your health and lengthen your life as well. Therefore, switching to a plant based diet is one of the best things you can do for yourself and your overall well-being.

People who consume plant-based products have a lower risk of developing diseases or having strokes because of the fiber, vitamins and minerals that come along with a plant-based diet. The fiber, vitamins and minerals, as well as healthy fats, are essential substances your body needs in order to function properly. Plant-based diet thus improve the blood lipid levels and better your brain health as well. There is a significant decrease in bad cholesterol in people who follow a plant-based diet.

It is never too late to change your diet! Whether you are 18, 36 or 50, it is still recommended to switch to a plant-based diet, as it is never too late to do so! These diets have quick and effective results that you will be noticing even after the first week of eating only plant-based meals. The first results you will notice will be the sense of accomplishment and satisfaction that comes with following a healthy diet. You will notice your mood has improved, in addition to not feel heavy after a meal, but instead feeling full and satisfied and yet energetic. After a period of following a plant-based diet, you will begin to notice the health benefits of doing so.

Your health-related problems will be reduced and you will feel a significant relief in terms of pains or discomfort you have been having.

What is important to know when switching to a plant-based diet is that you are not going to be on any kind of deprivation diet. Many people relate plant-based diet as a diet where you are depriving yourself of meat and dairy. However, when you switch to a plant-based diet you will not feel like you are missing anything, since your taste will adapt to your new eating habits. This will lead to you finding foods delicious that you maybe even disliked before. The human body is adapting constantly to the different inputs, and after a while, plant-based food will feel tasty and natural to you. The foods prepared of the healthy, nutritional ingredients are very delicious, especially if you follow the right recipes. Stick through this diet guide to learn some great plant based diet recipes you can include in your transition program. Once you see the benefits of the plant based diet and try some of the specialties, you will never want to go back to your eating habits again.

Transitioning from a meat to a plant based diet is not as difficult as everyone thinks. You can do it gradually, by increasing your fruit and vegetable intake while decreasing your meat and dairy intake. Minimizing meat consumption at first will make the transition seem effortless later, as you don't have to introduce drastic changes immediately. Instead of meat and dairy, you should start consuming the following foods:

- fruits such as apples, bananas, grapes, etc.
- vegetables such as kale, lettuce, peppers, corn, etc.
- tubers such as potatoes, beets, carrots, etc.
- whole grains such as rice, oats, millet, whole wheat, etc.
- legumes such as kidney beans, black beans, chickpeas, etc.

Therefore, your diet will be based on fruits, vegetables, tubers, whole grains and legumes. You can start implementing these changes by replacing meat in your favorite recipes and dishes with mushrooms or beans. Gradually, you will completely lose the habit of consuming meat and switch to a full plant based diet. To help your transition process, you should add more calories of legumes, whole grains and vegetables to your everyday routine, as that will make you feel full and thus reduce your desire to eat meat and dairy.

As soon as you start switching your diet you will notice how positively your body reacts to receiving all the nutrients it needs to function properly. The foods you should be focusing on include beans, that is, all legumes, berries, broccoli, cabbage, collards, nuts and kale.

Before we get into the detailed, 4 week program for switching to a plant based diet, here are a few tips that will help you make the transition easily.

- Include fruits and vegetables in every meal of the day. Instead of snacking on chocolate bars, switch to fruit or nutritional bars. Remember, an apple a day keeps the doctor away!
- Downsize your meat servings gradually. Put less meat on your plate and more veggies. Make sure that the ¾ of the plate consists of plant-based ingredients!

You can slowly transition by introducing two or three meat-free days to your week plan. As time goes by you will get used to this system and you will be able to skip meat more often, until fully switching to the plant based diet.

In addition to the many medical benefits of switching to a plant-based diet, there are also some truly powerful and indisputable cosmetic benefits as well. Many studies have shown that there is a significant and strong link between the consumption of dairy products like milk, butter, or cheese, and undesirable skin conditions like acne, eczema, and early signs of aging.

Milk contains many similar properties to the hormone testosterone due to other hormones like progesterone making their way into the milk. It is thought that these hormones stimulate the oil glands of the skin, especially the face. An excess of sebum, or oil, is produced and thus acne occurs. This excess oil clogs your pores and can lead to other troublesome skin blemishes such as blackheads and whiteheads. This continuous cycle of clogged pores, blemishes, and acne takes a lot out of your skin and can cause scarring and stress. This can lead to signs of premature aging and skin loses its elasticity and vitality. Many people who switch to a plant-based diet notice an incredibly rapid improvement in the condition of their skin. People who have suffered from acne and started eating plant-based foods have noticed their skin clear significantly. This is in no way by chance. Cutting out or greatly reducing dairy can really help give your skin a new lease on life. If you are struggling with acne and have tried nearly everything under the sun such as harsh chemicals, expensive facials and skin treatments, or countless different brands claiming to heal your skin problems,

something as simple as a plant-based diet may be the answer you've been searching for.

Followers of a plant-based diet have also raved about the excellent anti-aging benefits of the diet. Collagen, something our bodies naturally produce in abundance when we are young, is the key factor of what makes skin supple, resilient, firm, and have elasticity. As we get older, collagen production slows and our skin suffers as a result, becoming prone to sagginess and thinness. While this is a natural and inevitable part of life, collagen loss does not have to be so drastic as we age. A plant-based diet has been proven to boost collagen in your body by providing all of the important nutrients and amino acids that make up collagen and how it is produced. In a sense, subscribing to a plant-based diet is kind of like taking a dip in the fountain of youth! Fruits and vegetables like kale, broccoli, asparagus, spinach, grapefruit, lemons, and oranges are chock-full of vitamin C which is an extremely important component in producing the amino acids that make up collagen. The kind of lean protein found in nuts is important in keeping collagen around, adding to skin cell longevity and resilience. Red vegetables like tomatoes, beets, and red peppers all contain lycopene which is a kind of antioxidant that protects skin from the sun while simultaneously increases collagen production. Foods rich in zinc such as certain seeds and whole grains also promote collagen because the mineral repairs damaged cells and reduces inflammation. So many of the plant-based staples contain incredible amounts of all these collagen-boosting nutrients that you do not even have to go out of your way to seek them out. It is all right there in front of you! Looking and feeling younger has never been so easy. It really does start with the internal to make the external radiant and glowing, outer beauty starts from within.

In short, there are no two ways about it - switching to a plant based diet is good for your heart, your health, your mind, and even your physical appearance! The facts of the matter are undeniable. Plant foods contain so many of the incredibly good nutrients that our bodies need to function properly. Making these foods a priority and centering your meals around them rather than just eating vegetables as an occasional side dish or a piece of fruit every now and then makes a huge difference in your health. By eating a diet heavy on meat, dairy, and other animal products and processed foods, it is easy to miss out on the wonderfully beneficial vitamins, minerals, antioxidants, and other nutrients that are in fruits, vegetables, legumes, tubers, grains, nuts, and seeds. Switching to a plant-based diet gives you the opportunity to obtain all of these healthful ingredients that will without a doubt lead you to a better, more fulfilling life.

Weight Loss and better healthy

Individuals who have been eating a plant-based diet will argue that the meal plan is more than just a diet. It is a lifestyle. The mere fact that a plant-based diet aids in fighting off diseases means that it gives you an opportunity to live and enjoy life. Truth be told, our bodies are remarkable machines.

Nonetheless, they need to be taken care of by eating the right foods. Staying on a plant-only diet not only keeps your strong today, but it also ensures that you live longer. The exciting thing is that the diet is not complicated at all. You don't have to go through a lot of stress to maintain a plant-only diet. In addition, it is affordable. By making it a habit, you can take advantage of the many benefits of a plant-based diet, which we will explore below.

Did you know that over 69% of the adult population in the United States is obese (Kubala, 2018)? This is a worrying statistic as it means that more than half of the adult population is suffering. Additionally, they face the risk of suffering from hypertension and other cardiovascular diseases. Fortunately, there is a remedy to this. Simply changing your lifestyle and your diet can promote weight loss. That's not all; your overall health will also improve.

Plant-based diets have shown that they can aid in considerable weight loss due to their rich fiber content. The absence of processed foods in these diets also provides a huge boost in shedding those pounds.

A plant-only diet will also ensure that you don't gain weight in the long term. Unfortunately, numerous weight loss plans out there only help people in the short term, and individuals end up gaining more weight when they fail to stick to the weight loss plans. Therefore, with regard to sustainability, a plant-only diet is an ideal option.

Good digestion calls for plenty of fiber. The good news is that plants offer sufficient fiber to facilitate good digestion. It is vital to understand that you cannot just start eating tons of vegetables and fruits without a plan. If you are starting this diet, you should start slow. Your body needs ample time to adjust. Therefore, you should introduce your new diet slowly to prevent constipation, since most of it is composed of fiber.

One major problem with meat diets, processed foods, and dairy products is that they increase the risk of suffering from chronic illnesses like cancer, heart disease, and diabetes. The world today is fighting off these diseases by encouraging people to embrace healthy living through eating right and exercising. Plant-based diets are a healthy alternative as they lower the chances of suffering from these diseases.

Simply put, plant-only diets are heart healthy. This is a notable benefit of such diets. Nevertheless, it should be made clear that the type and quality of foods chosen matter greatly. There are some plant-based diets that can be considered unhealthy. For instance, shopping for and consuming processed fruits and vegetables that have a high sugar content will have a negative effect on the health of your heart. Therefore, it is imperative for a dieter to stick to recommended foods when opting for a plant-only diet.

Studies have also proven that plant-based diets can assist in lowering the risk of certain types of cancer. A research study conducted on over 69,000 individuals showed that vegan diets faced a reduced risk of gastrointestinal cancer, more so than those who maintained an ovo-vegetarian diet (Kubala, 2018).

Cognitive decline is not a new term to the elderly in our society.

A good number of aging individuals in our communities have to deal with their declining cognitive abilities. Often, we sympathize with them while forgetting that growing old is inevitable. We shouldn't just pity them; we should work towards maintaining a healthy society by eating right. Plant-only diets have shown to help in slowing down or preventing Alzheimer's disease and cognitive decline in the elderly population (Kubala, 2018). Antioxidants and plant compounds present in plant-based diets are effective in preventing Alzheimer's disease from progressing.

This is yet another common chronic disease that is robbing people of their loved ones. According to the World Health Organization, the number of people living with diabetes has risen from 108 million in 1980 to 422 million in 2014. This is attributed to unhealthy lifestyles and poor eating habits that people have adopted. Fortunately, diabetes is treatable, and its negative effects can be adequately prevented with the right diet. Of course, combining this with regular exercise helps even more.

Sticking to a plant-only diet will assist in enhancing your blood sugar control. As a result, you can ensure that you can effectively manage the disease if you are already suffering from it.

Minerals and vitamins are good sources of energy for the body. Plants are not only rich in them, but also contain phytonutrients, antioxidants, proteins, and healthy fats. All of these are essential nutrients for your brain. In addition, they are easy to digest, which makes it easy for the body to obtain energy from them.

We all know people who try every skin product imaginable just to get clear, smooth skin. What these people fail to understand is that how we look is more or less dictated by our food choices. Consequently, plant-based diets have a higher chance of providing your skin with the nutrients it needs to stay healthy. For instance, tomatoes provide the body with lycopene. This component safeguards the skin from sun damage. Sweet potatoes are known to provide us with vitamin C. The production of collagen will help your skin glow and encourage fast healing.

Chapter 3: What to Eat and What to Avoid

What to eat

Now that I talk of plant-focused foods, let's count the many options that you can enjoy.

● **Fruits**

All fruits are permitted on the plant-based diet and they can be enjoyed either fresh, frozen, or sun-dried. Eat the wide range of citrus fruits, berries, grapes, apples, melons, bananas, peaches, apricots, avocado, kiwi fruits, etc.

● **Vegetables**

A healthful plant-based sits in a wide range of vegetables. All vegetables are welcomed on the diet both above the ground and under the ground vegetables. Meanwhile, vegetables provide a wide range of vitamins and minerals.

Enjoy spinach, kale, mustard greens, collard greens, broccoli, cauliflower, asparagus, green beans, eggplants, carrots, tomatoes, bell peppers, zucchinis, beetroot, parsnips, turnips, potatoes, etc.

● **Legumes**

Legumes are an excellent source for plant-based protein and fiber. Fiber is one nutrient that many people lack; hence, it is necessary to consume foods like legumes often to enrich the body with enough fiber.

Eat the wide range of beans, chickpeas, lentils, peas, etc.

●**Whole Grains**

These are also fantastic for fiber sourcing and help maintain stable blood sugar. They are also rich in essential minerals like selenium, copper, and magnesium.

It is important to note that whole grains vary from bleached grains, therefore avoid processed flours, rice, pasta, and breads on the plant-based diet.

Eat brown rice, whole-wheat pasta, whole-grain bread, oats, barley, buckwheat, rye, quinoa, spelt, corn, etc.

●**Nuts and Nut Butters**

Nuts are an essential source of selenium, vitamin E, and plant-based protein. They are excellent additions to smoothies, puddings, desserts, and snacks.

Crunch on almonds, pecans, walnuts, macadamia nuts, hazelnuts, pistachios, cashew nuts, peanuts, brazil, etc.

● **Seeds**

Incorporate seeds into soups, snacks, smoothies, desserts, etc. They are rich in calcium, Vitamin E, and are a good source of healthy fats.

Consume flaxseeds, pepitas (pumpkin seeds), sunflower seeds, chia seeds, hemp seeds, sesame seeds, etc.

●**Healthy Oils and Fats**

Fats do not have to come from animal sources only. Some plant foods equally provide excellent fats for frying, searing, baking, and act as replacement for most dairy products. Meanwhile, they are rich in omega-3 fatty acids.

Use olive oil, avocados, canola oil, walnuts, peanuts, hemp seeds, flaxseeds, chia seeds, cashew nuts, coconut oil, etc.

●**Plant-Based Milk, Cream, and Cheeses**

Going plant-based doesn't mean starving yourself off creamy, milky, cheesy foods. You can enjoy plant-based alternatives of pasta alfredo, cheesecakes, etc.

Enjoy almond milk, soymilk, coconut milk, coconut cream, rice milk, cashew milk, cashew cream, hemp milk, oats milk, etc.

●Plant-Based Meats

Also, enrich your foods with meats options made from plant sources like soymilk and whole grains.

Eat tofu, tempeh, seitan, etc.

●Spices, Herbs, and Condiments

Nothing beats the preparation of foods than the aroma that exudes while cooking. Therefore, all ranges of homemade spices, herbs, and condiments are welcomed.

Use basil, parsley, rosemary, oregano, thyme, sage, marjoram, turmeric, curry, black pepper, salt, salsa, soy sauce, nutritional yeast, vinegar, homemade BBQ sauce, homemade plant-based mayonnaise, etc.

● Beverages

Coffee, sparking water, tea, smoothies, etc. are fine to drink.

Foods to avoid

For sticking to whole-foods on the plant-based diet, it is essential to eliminate animal products entirely. Also, avoid eating the following foods:

● Processed foods – prefer to use homemade unprocessed versions.

● Excess salt – many salt brands are highly processed while excess salt intake increases high blood pressure. Reduce your salt intake.

● Refined white carbohydrates – like white rice, white bread, white pasta.

● Sugary foods – swap them for fresh fruits, smoothies, freshly squeezed juices, etc. Avoid store-bought cakes, biscuits, pastries, soda, artificially flavored drinks, etc.

● Processed vegan and vegetarian alternatives that may include high amounts of salt and sugar.

● Greasy, fatty, and deep-fried foods – work with little amounts of fats as much as possible.

Macronutrients

Your body is transitioning in this diet as well. If you're not watching your intake, you may end up deficient in one or many things and this will harm your health. You can even go through what is called the keto flu. The keto flu is what happens when your body begins adjusting to running on a different ratio of macronutrients than it used to. You begin to experience flu-like symptoms and experience stomach pain, dizziness, brain fog, diarrhea, constipation, muscle cramps, trouble sleeping, sugar cravings, the inability to stay asleep, or lack of focus and concentration. This doesn't happen to everyone, but it is something to be aware of.

Vegans need calcium and vitamin D especially. Calcium is vital for maintaining strong bones and teeth. As you're still eating and consuming dairy foods on this diet, you will be able to get calcium into your system pretty easily. Greens are also a good source of calcium. Broccoli and kale are really good examples. Another is turnips and collard greens. Just remember what veggies are best for the ketogenic diet as well. In a ketogenic diet during the early stages when you're losing more calcium (because of the transitioning process where you're losing electrolytes), you will need more amounts of calcium as you're losing that too.

Vitamin D is also good for bone health. Since milk is high in both sugar and carbs and not good for ketogenic, you should try to find your vitamin D in cereal if you can.

If you're still not getting enough vitamin D and you don't get out in the sun much, you will probably need a supplement to help you get the right amount. They offer plant derived ones as well which is essential in a vegan diet where you do not use anything derived from animals.

Vitamin B12 or cyanocobalamin is necessary to produce red blood cells. This vitamin is important because it forms the red blood cells in your body. It also helps with the fatty acids in your body by breaking them down to produce vital energy that you will be able to use throughout your day. It's the most well-known B vitamin for a reason. It is also helpful with mental clarity and used to prevent anemia. Anemia is a condition that happens when you have a red blood cell deficiency or a deficiency of hemoglobin in the blood. This results in weariness and pallor. Pallor means you have an unhealthy pale appearance. So vitamin D is going to be a big issue if you're not getting enough as anemia can cause an entire host of problems. On a vegan ketogenic diet, you don't get very much leeway here. Eggs and milk both contain B12. It is not generally found in plant foods, but you can find it in fortified breakfast cereals. The problem is you can't have dairy. This means you would be finding it in your fortified cereals but that would not be enough for a vegan. If you find that you are not getting the amount that you need with these foods, you will need to find a supplement to correct it.

Zinc is important because it has a part in the formations of the proteins in your body as well as playing a role in cell division. It also has a part to play as an elemental part of the enzymes that are inside you. Zinc is more easily absorbed from animal products, but it can be absorbed from plant sources as well, though just not quite as easily. For a plant source of zinc, you've got choices from whole grains, wheat germ, soy products, and nuts.

Most nuts are high in carbs though, so you might not want to choose that option unless you're willing to possibly go too high in carbohydrates.

Micronutrients

Nutrients and micronutrients are going to be really important for you in this lifestyle because missing out on them can make you really sick and cause deficiencies in your body that would need to be corrected right away. The deficiencies can cause some serious issues and in some cases, life-threatening issues.

Micronutrients are nutrients that are needed for the human body. You usually need these in trace amounts. These micronutrients are part of development and growth. This is normal for the human body. This includes minerals, fatty acids, antioxidants, trace elements, and vitamins. Micronutrients your body protect itself from getting sick or help fight off diseases. These also ensure that the parts of your body under its care are being protected and functioning the way they're supposed to. This is a definite plus since these are in charge of almost every system in your body. Macronutrients, on the other hand, is a substance that is required in relatively large amounts by living organisms. Another way of describing it would be a type of food like a protein, fat, or carbs that are required in large amounts in the human diet.

A perfect example is processed food. Take cookies for example. A popular brand contains virtually zero micronutrients. Instead, it's mainly composed of carbohydrates, meaning, it's something to steer clear of on a ketogenic diet. They can also drastically spike your blood sugar. On the other side of this spectrum, foods such as leafy greens that you can consume on this diet are a great way to get your micronutrients. These include vitamin A, omega threes, and potassium.

The reason that you're making sure of getting the essential vitamins is that on the ketogenic diet, it can be low in micros if you are only trying to hit certain goals and not all of them.

One thing to remember is that you need both your micronutrients and macronutrients. You still need micronutrients and its value in your diet. Knowing how to compose meals that are rich in nutrients is important and will be a key factor in this diet and vegetables are really going to help you get it in as these are full of them.

Chapter 4: 31 Days meal plan

Day 1
Breakfast-Delicious Quiche made with
Cauliflower & Chickpea
Lunch- Grilled AHLT
Dinner- Sweet Potato Patties

Day 2
Breakfast- Tasty Oatmeal and Carrot Cake
Lunch- Loaded Black Bean Pizza
Dinner- Simple Sesame Stir-Fry

Day 3
Breakfast- Go-Green Smoothie
Lunch- Falafel Wrap
Dinner- Spaghetti and Buckwheat Meatballs

Day 4
Breakfast- Tasty Oatmeal Muffins
Lunch- Pad Thai Bowl
Dinner- Orange Walnut Pasta

Day 5
Breakfast- Glory Muffins
Lunch- Curry Spiced Lentil Burgers
Dinner- Roasted Cauliflower Tacos

Day 6
Breakfast- Amazing Almond & Banana
Granola
Lunch- Black Bean Taco Salad Bowl
Dinner- Build Your Own Mushroom Fajitas

Day 7
Breakfast- Pomegranate Overnight Oats
Lunch- Bibimbap Bowl
Dinner- Sun-dried Tomato and Pesto Quinoa

Day 8
Breakfast- Almond Chia Pudding
Lunch- Miso-Coconut Dragon Bowl
Dinner- Olive and White Bean Pasta

Day 9
Breakfast- Breakfast Parfait Popsicles
Lunch- Cashew-Ginger Soba Noodle Bowl
Dinner- Vietnamese Summer Rolls

Day 10
Breakfast- Apple Chia Pudding
Lunch- Mediterranean Hummus Pizza
Dinner- Potato Skin Samosas

Day 11
Breakfast- Pumpkin Spice Bites
Lunch- Curried Mango Chickpea Wrap
Dinner-Potato Skin Samosas

Day 12
Breakfast- Peach Quinoa Porridge
Lunch- Maple Dijon Burgers
Dinner-Sun-dried Tomato and Pesto Quinoa

Day 13
Breakfast- Chive Waffles with Mushrooms
Lunch- Cajun Burger
Dinner- Spicy Chickpea Sushi Rolls

Day 14
Breakfast- Lemon Spelt Scones
Lunch- Falafel Wrap
Dinner- Spaghetti and Buckwheat Meatballs

Day 15
Breakfast- Veggie Breakfast Scramble
Lunch- Bibimbap Bowl
Dinner- Sun-dried Tomato and Pesto Quinoa

Day 16
Breakfast- Strawberry Smoothie Bowl
Lunch- Curry Spiced Lentil Burgers
Dinner- Roasted Cauliflower Tacos

Day 17
Breakfast- Go-Green Smoothie
Lunch- Falafel Wrap
Dinner- Spaghetti and Buckwheat Meatballs

Day 18
Breakfast- Tasty Oatmeal Muffins
Lunch- Pad Thai Bowl
Dinner- Orange Walnut Pasta

Day 19
Breakfast- Glory Muffins
Lunch- Curry Spiced Lentil Burgers
Dinner- Roasted Cauliflower Tacos

Day 20
Breakfast- Amazing Almond & Banana
Granola
Lunch- Black Bean Taco Salad Bowl
Dinner- Build Your Own Mushroom Fajitas

Day 21
Breakfast- Pomegranate Overnight Oats
Lunch- Bibimbap Bowl
Dinner- Sun-dried Tomato and Pesto Quinoa

Day 22
Breakfast- Almond Chia Pudding
Lunch- Miso-Coconut Dragon Bowl
Dinner- Olive and White Bean Pasta

Day 23

Breakfast- Breakfast Parfait Popsicles
Lunch- Cashew-Ginger Soba Noodle Bowl
Dinner- Vietnamese Summer Rolls

Day 24
Breakfast- Apple Chia Pudding
Lunch- Mediterranean Hummus Pizza
Dinner- Potato Skin Samosas

Day 25
Breakfast- Pumpkin Spice Bites
Lunch- Curried Mango Chickpea Wrap
Dinner-Potato Skin Samosas

Day 26
Breakfast- Peach Quinoa Porridge
Lunch- Maple Dijon Burgers
Dinner-Sun-dried Tomato and Pesto Quinoa

Day 27
Breakfast- Chive Waffles with Mushrooms
Lunch- Cajun Burger

Dinner- Spicy Chickpea Sushi Rolls

Day 28
Breakfast- Lemon Spelt Scones
Lunch- Falafel Wrap
Dinner- Spaghetti and Buckwheat Meatballs

Day 29
Breakfast- Veggie Breakfast Scramble
Lunch- Bibimbap Bowl
Dinner- Sun-dried Tomato and Pesto Quinoa

Day 30
Breakfast- Strawberry Smoothie Bowl
Lunch- Curry Spiced Lentil Burgers
Dinner- Roasted Cauliflower Tacos

Day 31
Breakfast- Lemon Spelt Scones
Lunch- Falafel Wrap
Dinner- Spaghetti and Buckwheat Meatballs

Chapter 5: Breakfast Recipes

Delicious Quiche made with Cauliflower & Chickpea

Total time: 45 minutes
Ingredients
½ teaspoon of salt
1 cup of grated cauliflower
1 cup of chickpea flour
½ teaspoon of baking powder
½ zucchini, thinly sliced into half moons
1 tablespoon of flax meal
1 cup of water
1 freshly chopped sprig of fresh rosemary
½ teaspoon of Italian seasoning
½ freshly sliced red onion
¼ teaspoon of baking powder
Directions
In a bowl, combine all the dry ingredients.
Chop the onion and zucchini.
Grate the cauliflower so that it has a rice-like consistency, and add it to the dry ingredients. Now, add the water and mix well.
Add the zucchini, onion, and rosemary last. You will have a clumpy and thick mixture, but you should be able to spoon it into a tin.
You can use either a silicone or a metal cake tin with a removable bottom. Now put the mixture in the tin and press it down gently.
The top should be left messy to resemble a rough texture.
Bake at 350o F for about half an hour. You will know your quiche is ready when the top is golden.
You can serve the quiche warm or cold, as per your preference.

Tasty Oatmeal and Carrot Cake

Total time: 20 minutes
Ingredients
1 cup of water
½ teaspoon of cinnamon
1 cup of rolled oats
Salt
¼ cup of raisins
½ cup of shredded carrots
1 cup of non-dairy milk
¼ teaspoon of allspice
½ teaspoon of vanilla extract
Toppings:
¼ cup of chopped walnuts
2 tablespoons of maple syrup
2 tablespoons of shredded coconut
Directions
Put a small pot on low heat and bring the non-dairy milk, oats, and water to a simmer.
Now, add the carrots, vanilla extract, raisins, salt, cinnamon and allspice. You need to simmer all of the ingredients, but do not forget to stir them. You will know that they are ready when the liquid is fully absorbed into all of the ingredients (in about 7-10 minutes).
Transfer the thickened dish to bowls. You can drizzle some maple syrup on top or top them with coconut or walnuts.
This nutritious bowl will allow you to kickstart your day.

Go-Green Smoothie

Total time: 10 minutes
Ingredients
2 tablespoons of natural cashew butter
1 ripe frozen banana
2/3 cup of unsweetened coconut, soy, or almond milk
1 large handful of kale or spinach
Directions
Put everything inside a powerful blender.
Blend until you have a smooth, creamy shake.
Enjoy your special green smoothie.

Tasty Oatmeal Muffins

Total time: 30 minutes
Ingredients
½ cup of hot water
½ cup of raisins
¼ cup of ground flaxseed
2 cups of rolled oats
¼ teaspoon of sea salt
½ cup of walnuts
¼ teaspoon of baking soda
1 banana
2 tablespoons of cinnamon
¼ cup of maple syrup
Directions
Whisk the flaxseed with water and allow the mixture to sit for about 5 minutes.
In a food processor, blend all the ingredients along with the flaxseed mix. Blend everything for 30 seconds, but do not create a smooth substance. To create rough-textured cookies, you need to have a semi-coarse batter.
Put the batter in cupcake liners and place them in a muffin tin. As this is an oil-free recipe, you will need cupcake liners. Bake everything for about 20 minutes at 350 degrees.
Enjoy the freshly-made cookies with a glass of warm milk.

Glory Muffins

Total time: 30 minutes
Ingredients
1¾ cups flour
½ teaspoon baking powder
½ cup sugar
2 teaspoons cinnamon
½ teaspoon ground ginger
3 flax eggs
1 cup plant-based milk
½ cup maple syrup
1 teaspoon vanilla extract
1 apple, shredded
2 carrots, shredded
1 teaspoon baking soda
⅓ cup walnuts, chopped
½ teaspoon salt
Directions
The oven should be preheated at 350 degrees F.
Mix flaxseed with water in a bowl and leave for 10 minutes.
In a bowl, mix flour, sugar, ginger, cinnamon, baking soda, salt, and baking powder.
Stir in vanilla, maple syrup, and milk along with flaxseed mix.
Mix well to make a batter then fold in apple, nuts, and carrots.
Line a muffin tin with 6 muffin cups and divide the carrot batter evenly between the cups.
Bake for 20 minutes then serve.

Amazing Almond & Banana Granola

Total time: 75 minutes
Ingredients:
2 peeled and chopped ripe bananas
8 cups of rolled oats
1 teaspoon of salt
2 cups of freshly pitted and chopped dates
1 cup of slivered and toasted almonds
1 teaspoon of almond extract
Directions
Preheat the oven to 275o F.
Line two 13 x 18-inch baking sheets with parchment paper.
In a medium saucepan, add 1 cup of water and the dates, and bring to a boil. On medium heat, cook them for about 10 minutes. The dates will be soft and pulpy. Keep on adding water to the saucepan so that the dates do not stick to the pan.
After removing the dates from the heat, allow them to cool before you blend them with salt, almond extract, and bananas.
You will have a smooth and creamy puree.
Add this mixture to the oats, and give it a thorough mix.
Divide the mixture into equal halves and spread over the baking sheets.
Bake for about 30-40 minutes, stirring every 10 minutes or so.
You will know that the granola is ready when it becomes crispy.
After removing the baking sheets from the oven, allow them to cool. Then, add the slivered almonds.
You can store your granola in an airtight container and enjoy it whenever you are hungry.

Pomegranate Overnight Oats

Total time: 10 minutes
Ingredients
½ cup rolled oats
½ cup almond milk
½ cup pomegranate seeds
1 tablespoon ground flax seeds
1 tablespoon cocoa nibs
To Garnish:
¼ cup pomegranate seeds
2 teaspoon coconut shreds
Directions
In a sealable container, add everything and mix well.
Seal the container and refrigerate overnight.
Serve with coconut shreds and pomegranate seeds on top.

Almond Chia Pudding

Total time: 10 minutes
Ingredients
3 tablespoons almond butter
2 tablespoons maple syrup
1 cup almond milk
¼ cup plus 1 tablespoon chia seeds
Directions
In a sealable container, add everything and mix well.
Seal the container and refrigerate overnight.
Serve with a splash of almond milk.

Breakfast Parfait Popsicles

Total time: 10 minutes
Ingredients
1 cup soy yogurt
1 cup berries
1 cup granola
Directions
In a popsicle mold, divide the berries.
Add yogurt to the molds and gently mix the berries using a stick.
Sprinkle granola on top and place the popsicle sticks in the mixture.
Freeze overnight.
Serve.

Apple Chia Pudding

Total time: 15 minutes
Ingredients
Chia Pudding:
4 tablespoons chia seeds
1 cup almond milk
½ teaspoon cinnamon
Apple Pie Filling:
1 large apple, peeled, cored and chopped
¼ cup water
2 teaspoons maple syrup
Pinch cinnamon
2 tablespoons golden raisins
Directions
In a sealable container, add cinnamon, chia seeds and almond milk, mix well.
Seal the container and refrigerate overnight.
In a medium pot, combine all apple pie filling ingredients and cook for 5 minutes.
Serve the chia pudding with apple filling on top.
Enjoy.

Pumpkin Spice Bites

Total time: 10 minutes
Ingredients
½ cup pumpkin puree
½ cup almond butter
¼ cup maple syrup
1 teaspoon pumpkin pie spice
1⅓ cup rolled oats
⅓ cup pumpkin seeds
⅓ cup raisins
2 tablespoons chia seeds
Directions
In a sealable container, add everything and mix well.
Seal the container and refrigerate overnight.
Roll the mixture into small balls.
Serve.

Chive Waffles with Mushrooms

Total time: 35 minutes
Ingredients
2 cups soy milk
1 teaspoon apple cider vinegar
2 tablespoon rapeseed oil
⅓ cup cooked, mashed sweet potato
5 ounces polenta
5 ounces plain flour
1 tablespoon baking powder
1 small bunch chives, chopped
1 tablespoon maple syrup
2 teaspoons light soy sauce
6 large mushrooms, sliced
Olive oil, for frying
Soy yogurt, to serve
Directions
Preheat your waffle iron.
Meanwhile, sauté mushrooms with salt and black pepper in a suitable pan.
Keep the mushrooms aside ready to serve.
In a bowl, mash sweet potato and stir in the rest of the ingredients.
Mix it well to make the waffle batter.
Pour batter into the waffle iron until it is filled and close it to cook for 5 minutes.
Make 5 more waffles using this batter.
Serve with the sautéed mushrooms and yogurt on top.

Lemon Spelt Scones

Total time: 28 minutes
Ingredients
1¾ cups spelt flour
1¼ cup whole spelt
⅔ cup coconut sugar
2 teaspoons baking powder
½ teaspoon salt
3 tablespoons lemon zest
½ cup coconut oil
1 cup coconut cream
2 tablespoons almond milk
2 cups frozen raspberries
Directions
Preheat your oven to 425 degrees F.
Whisk dry ingredients in a stand mixer using whisk attachment.
Freeze the dry mixture for 10 minutes then place it back on the mixer.
Using the paddle attachment, stir in coconut oil, coconut cream, and almond milk then beat until smooth.
Fold in frozen raspberries and mix again, divide the dough into two parts.
Spread each part into a thick disk and cut each into 6 wedges of equal size.
Line a suitable baking sheet with parchment paper and place the wedges on the tray.
Bake for 18 minutes then serve.

Veggie Breakfast Scramble

Total time: 24 minutes
Ingredients
1 cup yellow onions, chopped
1 cup red bell peppers, diced
1½ cups zucchini, sliced
3 cups cauliflower florets
1 tablespoon garlic, minced
1 tablespoon tamari
2 tablespoons vegetable broth
2 tablespoons nutritional yeast
1 (15 ounce) can chickpeas, drained
2 cups baby spinach, chopped
Spice Mix:
1 teaspoon onion powder
1 teaspoon garlic powder
1 teaspoon dried minced onions
¾ teaspoon dried ground mustard powder
1 teaspoon dried thyme leaves
1 teaspoon smoked paprika
¼ teaspoon turmeric
¾ teaspoon salt
¼ teaspoon black pepper
Directions
In a suitable pan, add cooking oil and all the vegetables.
Cook while stirring for 7 minutes on medium heat.
Toss in the chickpeas and all the spices.
Continue sautéing for another 7 minutes.
Serve warm.

Strawberry Smoothie Bowl

Total time: 30 minutes
Ingredients
Smoothie bowl:
1 banana frozen
1½ cups frozen strawberries
½ cup coconut milk
Toppings:
Fresh strawberries sliced
Fresh bananas sliced
Chia seeds
 Directions
In a blender jug, puree all the ingredients for the smooth bowl.
Pour the smoothie in the serving bowl.
Add strawberries, banana and chia seeds on top.
Chill well then serve.

Peanut Butter Granola

Total time: 57 minutes

Ingredients

Nonstick spray
4 cups oats
⅓ cup of cocoa powder
¾ cup peanut butter
⅓ cup maple syrup
⅓ cup avocado oil
1½ teaspoons vanilla extract
½ cup cocoa nibs
6 ounces dark chocolate, chopped

Directions

Preheat your oven to 300 degrees F.
Spray a baking sheet with cooking spray.
In a medium saucepan add oil, maple syrup, and peanut butter.
Cook for 2 minutes on medium heat, stirring.
Add the oats and cocoa powder, mix well.
Spread the coated oats on the baking sheet.
Bake for 45 minutes, occasionally stirring.
Garnish with dark chocolate, cocoa nibs, and peanut butter.
Serve.

Sweet Potato Toasts

Total time: 20 minutes

Ingredients

2 large sweet potatoes, sliced into ¼ inch thick slices
1 tablespoon avocado oil
1 teaspoon salt
½ cup guacamole
½ cup tomatoes, sliced

Directions

Preheat your oven to 425 degrees F.
Cover a baking sheet with parchment paper.
Rub the potato slices with oil and salt and place them on a baking sheet.
Bake for 5 minutes in the oven, then flip and bake again for 5 minutes.
Top the baked slices with guacamole and tomatoes.
Serve.

Tofu Scramble Tacos

Total time: 20 minutes
Ingredients
1 package tofu
¼ cup nutritional yeast
2 teaspoons garlic powder
2 teaspoons cumin
2 teaspoons chili powder
½ teaspoon turmeric
1 teaspoon salt
½ teaspoon pepper
1 tablespoon avocado oil
Warm corn tortillas
Directions
In a pan, add avocado oil and tofu.
Sauté and crumble the tofu on medium heat.
Stir in all the remaining spices and yeast.
Mix and cook for 2 minutes.
Serve on tortillas.

Omelet with Chickpea Flour

Total time: 30 minutes
Ingredients
½ teaspoon of onion powder
¼ teaspoon of black pepper
1 cup of chickpea flour
½ teaspoon of garlic powder
½ teaspoon of baking soda
¼ teaspoon of white pepper
1/3 cup of nutritional yeast
3 finely chopped green onions
4 ounces of sautéed mushrooms
Directions
In a small bowl, mix the onion powder, white pepper, chickpea flour, garlic powder, black and white pepper, baking soda, and nutritional yeast. Add 1 cup of water and create a smooth batter.

On medium heat, put a frying pan and add the batter just like the way you would cook pancakes. On the batter, sprinkle some green onion and mushrooms. Flip the omelet and cook evenly on both sides.

Once both sides are cooked, serve the omelet with spinach, tomatoes, hot sauce, and salsa. Enjoy a guilt-free meal.

A Toast to Remember

Total time: 25 minutes

Ingredients

1 can of black beans
Pinch of sea salt
2 pieces of whole-wheat toast
¼ teaspoon of chipotle spice
Pinch of black pepper
1 teaspoon of garlic powder
1 freshly juiced lime
1 freshly diced avocado
¼ cup of corn
3 tablespoons of finely diced onion
½ freshly diced tomato
Fresh cilantro

Directions

Mix the chipotle spice with the beans, salt, garlic powder, and pepper. Stir in the lime juice. Boil all of these until you have a thick and starchy mix.

In a bowl, mix the corn, tomato, avocado, red onion, cilantro, and juice from the rest of the lime. Add some pepper and salt.

Toast the bread and first spread the black bean mixture followed by the avocado mix.

Take a bite of wholesome goodness!

Onion & Mushroom Tart with a Nice Brown Rice Crust

Total time: 65 minutes

Ingredients

1 ½ pounds of mushrooms: button, portabella, or shiitake
1 cup of short-grain brown rice
2 ¼ cups of water
½ teaspoon of ground black pepper
2 teaspoons of herbal spice blend
1 sweet large onion
7 ounces of extra-firm tofu
1 cup of plain non-dairy milk
2 teaspoons of onion powder
2 teaspoons of low-sodium soy or tamari sauce
1 teaspoon of molasses
¼ teaspoon of ground turmeric
¼ cup of white wine or cooking sherry
¼ cup of tapioca or arrowroot powder

Directions

Cook the brown rice and put it aside for later use.

Slice the onions into thin strips and sauté them in water until they are soft. Then, add the molasses, and cook them for a few minutes.

Next, sauté the mushrooms in water with the herbal spice blend. Once the mushrooms are cooked and they are soft, add the white wine or sherry. Cook everything for a few more minutes.

In a blender, combine milk, tofu, arrowroot, turmeric, and onion powder till you have a smooth mixture

On a pie plate, create a layer of rice, spreading evenly to form a crust. The rice should be warm and not cold. It will be easy to work with warm rice. You can also use a pastry roller to get an even crust. With your fingers, gently press the sides.

Take half of the tofu mixture and the mushrooms and spoon them over the tart dish. Smooth the level with your spoon.

Now, top the layer with onions followed by the tofu mixture. You can smooth the surface again with your spoon. Sprinkle some black pepper on top.

Bake the pie at 350o F for about 45 minutes. Toward the end, you can cover it loosely with tin foil. This will help the crust to remain moist.

Allow the pie crust to cool down, so that you can slice it. If you are in love with vegetarian dishes, there is no way that you will not love this pie.

Perfect Breakfast Shake

Total time: 10 minutes

Ingredients

3 tablespoons of raw cacao powder
1 cup of soy/almond milk
2 frozen bananas
3 tablespoons of natural peanut butter

Directions

Use a powerful blender to combine all the ingredients.
Process everything until you have a smooth shake.
Enjoy a hearty shake to kickstart your day.

Perfect Polenta with a Dose of Cranberries & Pears

Total time: 15 minutes
Ingredients
2 pears freshly cored, peeled, and diced
1 batch of warm basic polenta
¼ cup of brown rice syrup
1 teaspoon of cinnamon
1 cup of dried or fresh cranberries
Directions
Warm the polenta in a medium-sized saucepan. Then, add the cranberries, pears, and cinnamon powder.
Cook everything, stirring occasionally. You will know that the dish is ready when the pears are soft.
The entire dish will be done within 10 minutes.
Divide the polenta equally among 4 bowls. Add some pear compote as the last finishing touch.
Now you can dig into this hassle-free breakfast bowl full of goodness.

Tempeh Bacon Smoked to Perfection

Total time: 45 minutes
Ingredients
3 tablespoons of maple syrup
8 ounce packages of tempeh
¼ cup of soy or tamari sauce
2 teaspoons of liquid smoke
Directions
In a steamer basket, steam the block of tempeh.
Mix the tamari, maple syrup, and liquid smoke in a medium-sized bowl.
Once the tempeh cools down, slice into stripes and add to the prepared marinade. Remember: the longer the tempeh marinates, the better the flavor will be. If possible, refrigerate overnight. If not, marinate for at least half an hour.
In a sauté pan, cook the tempeh on medium-high heat with a bit of the marinade.
Once the strips get crispy on one side, turn them over so that both sides are evenly cooked.
You can add some more marinade to cook the tempeh, but they should be properly caramelized. It will take about 5 minutes for each side to cook.
Enjoy the crispy caramelized tempeh with your favorite dip.

Breakfast Burritos

Total time: 20 minutes
Ingredients
2 (15 oz) cans black beans, drained and rinsed
½ cup of water
4 whole-wheat tortillas
8 leaves romaine lettuce
2 tomatoes, sliced
2 avocados, peeled, pitted, and sliced
1 ½ cups salsa
Seasonings:
1 tbsp garlic powder
1 tbsp onion powder
1 tbsp chili powder
1 tsp dried cumin
1 tsp dried oregano
Directions
In a medium-sized pot, add the beans, water, and seasonings. Allow boiling over medium heat and then simmer for 10 minutes. Drain the beans after.
Onto the whole wheat tortillas, add one or two leaves of romaine lettuce, tomatoes, and avocado.
Add the black beans on top and then, the salsa.
Serve the burritos immediately.

Gingerbread Chia Porridge

Total time: 25 minutes
Ingredients
¼ cup Chia Seeds
Pinch of Clove, grounded
¾ cup Soy Milk, unsweetened
¼ tsp. Cinnamon, grounded
1 tbsp. Maple Syrup
Dash of Sea Salt
¼ tsp. Ginger, grounded
For garnishing:
1 tbsp. Raisins
Directions
Start by combining all the ingredients needed to make the oatmeal in a mason jar.
Place the Mason jar in the refrigerator for 8 hours.
Stir once the porridge before keeping it for refrigeration.
Now, garnish it with raisins.
Serve and enjoy.

Protein Granola

Total time: 25 minutes
Ingredients
2 tbsp. Flax Seed, grounded
1/3 cup Chocolate Chips
¼ cup Almond Butter
1 tsp. Vanilla Extract
1 tsp. Cinnamon
¼ cup Agave Nectar
¼ tsp. Salt
2 cups Rolled Oats
Directions
For making this healthy granola, you first need to preheat the oven to 325 °F.
After that, melt almond butter and honey together in a small saucepan over medium-low heat.
Then, spoon in the agave nectar to it. Mix well.
Now, remove the pan from the heat. Spoon in the oats, cinnamon, flax seeds, and salt to it. Tip: Mix the mixture well so that the butter honey mixture coats the oats well.
Next, transfer the oats mixture to a parchment paper-lined baking sheet and spread it across evenly.
Bake for 8 minutes. Once eight minutes is up, pull out the sheet from the oven and stir it well.
After stirring, keep the pan in the oven and bake for further 8 minutes or until lightly golden.
Allow the mixture to cool completely. Spoon in the chocolate chips.
Serve and enjoy.

Almond TEff Porridge

Total time: 25 minutes
Ingredients
¼ tsp. Cinnamon, grounded
1 cup Whole Grain Teff
¼ cup Almonds, crushed
1 ½ cup Water
¼ tsp. Sea Salt
1 ½ cup Almond Milk, unsweetened
1 Banana, sliced
1 tbsp. Extra Virgin Olive Oil
Directions
First, place teff, banana slices, almond milk, sea salt, water, cinnamon, and coconut oil in a deep saucepan over medium heat.
Stir well and bring the teff mixture to a boil.
Once it starts boiling, lower the heat to low.
Then, cover the pan with a lid.
Next, allow the teff mixture to simmer for 15 to 20 minutes. Tip: Make sure to stir it continuously so that the teff doesn't stick to the bottom of the pan.
Take the saucepan from the heat once the teff gets cooked.
Finally, transfer to the serving bowl and enjoy.

Raspberry Overnight Oats

Total time: 5 minutes
Ingredients
1 tsp. Maple Syrup
¼ cup White Beans
¼ cup Raspberries
½ cup Rolled Oats
10 Almonds, raw & chopped
1 tsp. Chia Seeds
1 tsp. Maple Syrup
2/3 cup Soy Milk
Directions
To start with, place the beans in a large mason jar and mash it with a fork.
Next, stir in all the remaining ingredients to the Mason jar. Mix well.
Now, keep the jar in the refrigerator overnight.
In the morning, keep the Mason jar out of the refrigerator and mix well.
Serve immediately and enjoy it.

Coconut Buckwheat Porridge

Total time: 20 minutes
Ingredients
1 cup Water
2 tsp. Vanilla Extract
1 cup Buckwheat Grouts
Dash of Salt
¼ cup Chia Seeds
¼ tsp. Cinnamon
3 cups Coconut Milk, unsweetened
Dash of Salt
Directions
For making this high-protein oatmeal, you need to mix all the ingredients in a large mixing bowl until combined well.
Then, cover the bowl with plastic cling and place it in the refrigerator overnight.
Next morning, transfer the contents to a deep saucepan over medium heat.
Cook for 10 minutes or until thickened. Tip: Make sure to stir it continuously.
Serve it hot or warm.

Chickpea Scramble Bowl

Total time: 20 minutes
Ingredients
¼ of 1 Onion, diced
15 oz. Chickpeas
2 Garlic cloves, minced
½ tsp. Turmeric
½ tsp. Black Pepper
½ tsp. Extra Virgin Olive Oil
½ tsp. Salt
Directions
Begin by placing the chickpeas in a large bowl along with a bit of water.
Soak for few minutes and then mash the chickpeas lightly with a fork while leaving some of them in the whole form.
Next, spoon in the turmeric, pepper, and salt to the bowl. Mix well.
Then, heat oil in a medium-sized skillet over medium-high heat.
Once the oil becomes hot, stir in the onions.
Sauté the onions for 3 to 4 minutes or until softened.
Then, add the garlic and cook for further 1 minute or until aromatic.
After that, stir in the mashed chickpeas. Cook for another 4 minutes or until thickened.
Serve along with micro greens. Place the greens at the bottom, followed by the scramble, and top it with cilantro or parsley.

Maple Flavoured Oatmeal

Total time: 30 minutes
Ingredients
2 tbsp. Maple Syrup
1 cup Oatmeal
½ tsp. Cinnamon
2 ½ cup Water
2/3 cup Soy Milk
1 tsp. Earth Balance or Vegan Butter
Directions
To start with, place oatmeal and water in a medium-sized saucepan over medium-high heat.
Bring the mixture to a boil.
Next, lower the heat and cook for further 13 to 15 minutes while keeping the pan covered. Tip: At this point, all the water should get absorbed by the grains.
Now, remove the pan from the heat and fluff this mixture with a fork.
Cover the pan again. Set it aside for 5 minutes.
Then, stir in all the remaining ingredients to the oatmeal mixture until everything comes together.
Serve and enjoy.

Chocolate Chip Cookie Dough

Total time: 10 minutes
Ingredients
½ tsp. Sea Salt
2 cups Chickpeas, cooked & drained
¼ cup Maple Syrup
1/3 cup Coconut Oil, melted
3 tbsp. Coconut Flour
2 tsp. Vanilla Extract
Directions
To make this delightful cookie dough, first blend the chickpeas in a high-speed blender for a minute or until smooth.
Spoon in the oil, sea salt, maple syrup, and vanilla extract. Blend for a further minute or until combined.
Next, stir in the coconut flour and blend again. Scrape the sides.
Now, transfer the mixture to a medium-sized bowl and place in the refrigerator for 2 hours.
Serve on its own or with crackers.

Banana Strawberry Oats

Total time: 30 minutes
Ingredients
1 tbsp. Almonds, sliced
½ cup Oats
½ tsp. Cinnamon
1 cup Zucchini, shredded
½ of 1 Banana, mashed
1 cup Water
½ cup Strawberries, sliced
Dash of Sea Salt
1 tbsp. Flax Meal
½ scoop of Protein Powder
Directions
First, combine oats, salt, water, and zucchini in a large saucepan.
Cook the mixture over medium-high heat and cook for 8 to 10 minutes or until the liquid is absorbed.
Now, spoon in all the remaining ingredients to the mixture and give everything a good stir.
Finally, transfer the mixture to a serving bowl and top it with almonds and berries.
Serve and enjoy.

Chapter 6: Lunch Recipes

Grilled AHLT

Total time: 15 minutes
Ingredients
¼ cup Classic **Hummus**
2 slices whole-grain bread
¼ avocado, sliced
½ cup lettuce, chopped
½ tomato, sliced
Pinch sea salt
Pinch freshly ground black pepper
1 teaspoon olive oil, divided
Directions
1.Spread some hummus on each slice of bread. Then layer the avocado, lettuce, and tomato on one slice, sprinkle with salt and pepper, and top with the other slice.
2.Heat a skillet to medium heat, and drizzle ½ teaspoon of the olive oil just before putting the sandwich in the skillet. Cook for 3 to 5 minutes, then lift the sandwich with a spatula, drizzle the remaining ½ teaspoon olive oil into the skillet, and flip the sandwich to grill the other side for 3 to 5 minutes. Press it down with the spatula to seal the vegetables inside.
3.Once done, remove from the skillet and slice in half to serve.

Loaded Black Bean Pizza

Total time: 30 minutes
Ingredients
2 prebaked pizza crusts
½ cup Spicy Black Bean Dip
1 tomato, thinly sliced
Pinch freshly ground black pepper
1 carrot, grated
Pinch sea salt
1 red onion, thinly sliced
1 avocado, sliced
Directions
1.Preheat the oven to 400°F.
2.Lay the two crusts out on a large baking sheet. Spread half the Spicy Black Bean Dip on each pizza crust. Then layer on the tomato slices with a pinch pepper if you like.
3.Sprinkle the grated carrot with the sea salt and lightly massage it in with your hands. Spread the carrot on top of the tomato, then add the onion.
4.Pop the pizzas in the oven for 10 to 20 minutes, or until they're done to your taste.
5.Top the cooked pizzas with sliced avocado and another sprinkle of pepper.
Options: Try having this as a fresh unbaked pizza. Just toast a pita or bake the crust before loading it up, and perhaps use scallions instead of red. Bonus points—and flavor—if you top it with fresh alfalfa sprouts.

Falafel Wrap

Total time: 70 minutes
Ingredients
FOR THE FALAFEL PATTIES
1 (14-ounce) can chickpeas, drained and rinsed, or 1½ cups cooked
1 zucchini, grated
2 scallions, minced
¼ cup fresh parsley, chopped
2 tablespoons black olives, pitted and chopped (optional)
1 tablespoon tahini, or almond, cashew, or sunflower seed butter
1 tablespoon lemon juice, or apple cider vinegar
½ teaspoon ground cumin
¼ teaspoon paprika
¼ teaspoon sea salt
1 teaspoon olive oil (optional, if frying)
FOR THE WRAP
1 whole-grain wrap or pita
¼ cup Classic **Hummus**
½ cup fresh greens
1 baked falafel patty
¼ cup cherry tomatoes, halved
¼ cup diced cucumber
¼ cup chopped avocado, or **Guacamole**
¼ cup cooked quinoa, or **Tabbouleh Salad** (optional)

Directions for the falafel
1.Use a food processor to pulse the chickpeas, zucchini, scallions, parsley, and olives (if using) until roughly chopped. Just pulse—don't purée. Or use a potato masher to mash the chickpeas in a large bowl and stir in the grated and chopped veggies.
2.In a small bowl, whisk together the tahini and lemon juice, and stir in the cumin, paprika, and salt. Pour this into the chickpea mixture, and stir well (or pulse the food processor) to combine. Taste and add more salt, if needed. Using your hands, form the mix into 6 patties.
3.You can either panfry or bake the patties. To panfry, heat a large skillet to medium, add 1 teaspoon of olive oil, and cook the patties about 10 minutes on the first side. Flip, and cook another 5 to 7 minutes. To bake them, put them on a baking sheet lined with parchment paper and bake at 350°F for 30 to 40 minutes.

Directions for the wrap
1.Lay the wrap on a plate and spread the hummus down the center. Then lay on the greens and crumble the falafel patty on top. Add the tomatoes, cucumber, avocado, and quinoa.
2.Fold in both ends, and wrap up as tightly as you can. If you have a sandwich press, you can press the wraps for about 5 minutes. This will travel best in a reusable lunch box, or reusable plastic lunch wrap.

Pad Thai Bowl

Total time: 20 minutes
Ingredients
7 ounces brown rice noodles
1 teaspoon olive oil, or 1 tablespoon vegetable broth or water
2 carrots, peeled or scrubbed, and julienned
1 cup thinly sliced napa cabbage, or red cabbage
1 red bell pepper, seeded and thinly sliced
2 scallions, finely chopped
2 to 3 tablespoons fresh mint, finely chopped
1 cup bean sprouts
¼ cup Peanut Sauce
¼ cup fresh cilantro, finely chopped
2 tablespoons roasted peanuts, chopped
Fresh lime wedges
Directions
1.Put the rice noodles in a large bowl or pot, and cover with boiling water. Let sit until they soften, about 10 minutes. Rinse, drain, and set aside to cool.
2.Heat the oil in a large skillet to medium-high, and sauté the carrots, cabbage, and bell pepper until softened, 7 to 8 minutes. Toss in the scallions, mint, and bean sprouts and cook for just a minute or two, then remove from the heat.
3.Toss the noodles with the vegetables, and mix in the Peanut Sauce.
4.Transfer to bowls, and sprinkle with cilantro and peanuts. Serve with a lime wedge to squeeze onto the dish for a flavor boost.
Options: To enjoy an even more nutrient-dense version of this bowl, leave out the rice noodles and peel or spiralize a zucchini or carrot into long "noodles."

Curry Spiced Lentil Burgers

Total time: 80 minutes
Ingredients
1 cup lentils
2½ to 3 cups water
3 carrots, grated
1 small onion, diced
¾ cup whole-grain flour (see Options for gluten-free below)
1½ to 2 teaspoons curry powder
½ teaspoon sea salt
Pinch freshly ground black pepper
Directions
1.Put the lentils in a medium pot with the water. Bring to a boil and then simmer for about 30 minutes, until soft.
2.While the lentils are cooking, put the carrots and onion in a large bowl. Toss them with the flour, curry powder, salt, and pepper.
3.When the lentils are cooked, drain off any excess water, then add them to the bowl with the veggies. Use a potato masher or a large spoon to mash them slightly, and add more flour if you need to get the mixture to stick together. The amount of flour depends on how much water the lentils absorbed, and on the texture of the flour, so use more or less until the mixture sticks when you form it into a ball. Scoop up ¼-cup portions and form into 12 patties.
4.You can either panfry or bake the burgers. To panfry, heat a large skillet to medium, add a tiny bit of oil, and cook the burgers about 10 minutes on the first side. Flip, and cook another 5 to 7 minutes. To bake them, put them on a baking sheet lined with parchment paper and bake at 350°F for 30 to 40 minutes.
Options: For the whole-grain flour, use whatever flour you like. Sorghum, rice, oat, buckwheat, and even almond meal would work and make these gluten-free. The flour in this recipe is just a binding agent, so it can be any type.

Black Bean Taco Salad Bowl

Total time: 20 minutes

Ingredients

FOR THE BLACK BEAN SALAD

1 (14-ounce) can black beans, drained and rinsed, or 1½ cups cooked

1 cup corn kernels, fresh and blanched, or frozen and thawed

¼ cup fresh cilantro, or parsley, chopped

Zest and juice of 1 lime

1 to 2 teaspoons chili powder

Pinch sea salt

1½ cups cherry tomatoes, halved

1 red bell pepper, seeded and chopped

2 scallions, chopped

FOR 1 SERVING OF TORTILLA CHIPS

1 large whole-grain tortilla or wrap

1 teaspoon olive oil

Pinch sea salt

Pinch freshly ground black pepper

Pinch dried oregano

Pinch chili powder

FOR 1 BOWL

1 cup fresh greens (lettuce, spinach, or whatever you like)

¾ cup cooked quinoa, or brown rice, millet, or other whole grain

¼ cup chopped avocado, or **Guacamole**

¼ cup Fresh Mango Salsa

Directions for the black bean salad

Toss all the ingredients together in a large bowl.

Directions for the tortilla chips

Brush the tortilla with olive oil, then sprinkle with salt, pepper, oregano, chili powder, and any other seasonings you like. Slice it into eighths like a pizza. Transfer the tortilla pieces to a small baking sheet lined with parchment paper and put in the oven or toaster oven to toast or broil for 3 to 5 minutes, until browned. Keep an eye on them, as they can go from just barely done to burned very quickly.

Directions for the bowl

Lay the greens in the bowl, top with the cooked quinoa, ⅓ of the black bean salad, the avocado, and salsa.

Make ahead: The black bean mixture tastes better if you make it in advance, so the flavors have time to mix and mingle. Keep leftovers in the fridge in an airtight container.

Bibimbap Bowl

Total time: 30 minutes
Ingredients
½ cup cooked chickpeas
2 tablespoons tamari or soy sauce, divided
1 tablespoon plus 2 teaspoons toasted sesame oil, divided
¾ cup cooked brown rice, or quinoa, millet, or any other whole grain
1 teaspoon olive oil, or 1 tablespoon vegetable broth or water
1 carrot, scrubbed or peeled, and julienned
2 garlic cloves, minced, divided
Pinch sea salt
½ cup asparagus, cut into 2-inch pieces
½ cup chopped spinach
½ cup bean sprouts
3 tablespoons hot pepper paste (the Korean version is gochujang)
1 tablespoon toasted sesame seeds
1 scallion, chopped
Directions
1.In a small bowl, toss the chickpeas with 1 tablespoon tamari and 1 teaspoon toasted sesame oil. Set aside to marinate.
2.Put the cooked brown rice in a large serving bowl, so that you'll be ready to add the vegetables as they cook.
3.Heat the olive oil a large skillet over medium heat, and start by sautéing the carrot and 1 garlic clove with the salt. Once they've softened, about 5 minutes, remove them from the skillet and put them on top of the rice in one area of the bowl.
4.Next, sauté the asparagus, adding a bit more oil if necessary, and when soft, about 5 minutes, place next to the carrots in the bowl.
5.Add a bit of water to the skillet and quick steam the spinach with the other garlic clove, just until the spinach wilts. Drizzle with the remaining 1 tablespoon tamari and 1 teaspoon toasted sesame oil. Lay the spinach on the other side of the carrots in the bowl.
6.You could lightly sauté the bean sprouts if you wish, but they're nice raw. However you prefer them, add them to the bowl.
7.Place the marinated chickpeas in the final area of the bowl.
8.In a small bowl, mix together the hot pepper paste with 1 tablespoon sesame oil. Scoop that into the middle of the bowl. Sprinkle with sesame seeds and scallions, then mix it all together and enjoy!

Cashew-Ginger Soba Noodle Bowl

Total time: 25 minutes

Ingredients

FOR THE BOWLS

7 ounces soba noodles

1 carrot, peeled or scrubbed, and julienned

1 bell pepper, any color, seeded and thinly sliced

1 cup snow peas, or snap peas, trimmed and sliced in half

2 tablespoons chopped scallions

1 cup chopped kale, spinach, or lettuce

1 avocado, thinly sliced

2 tablespoons cashews, chopped

FOR THE DRESSING

1 tablespoon grated fresh ginger

2 tablespoons cashew butter, or almond or sunflower seed butter

2 tablespoons rice vinegar, or apple cider vinegar

2 tablespoons tamari, or soy sauce

1 teaspoon toasted sesame oil

2 to 3 tablespoons water (optional)

Directions

1.Boil a medium pot of water and add the noodles. Keep it at a low boil, turning down the heat and adding cool water if necessary to keep it just below a rolling boil. The soba will take 6 to 7 minutes to cook, and you can stir occasionally to make sure they don't stick to each other or the bottom of the pot. Once they're cooked, drain them in a colander and rinse with hot or cold water, depending on whether you want a hot or cold bowl.

2.You can have the vegetables raw, in which case you just need to cut them up. If you'd like to cook them, heat a skillet to medium-high, and sauté the carrot with a little water, broth, olive oil, or sesame oil. Once the carrot has softened slightly, add the bell pepper. Then add the peas and scallions, to warm for a minute, before turning off the heat.

3.Make the dressing by squeezing the grated ginger for its juice, then whisking together all the ingredients, or puréeing in a small blender, adding 2 to 3 tablespoons of water as needed to make a creamy consistency. Set aside.

4.Arrange your bowl, starting with a layer of chopped kale or spinach (for hot noodles) or lettuce (for cold noodles), then the noodles drizzled with some extra tamari, then the vegetables.

5.Top with the dressing, sliced avocado, and a sprinkle of chopped cashews.

Make ahead: Cooked and rinsed soba noodles keep well in the fridge, so make a whole package and keep them on hand for quick weeknight bowls or lunches to go.

Mediterranean Hummus Pizza

Total time: 40 minutes
Ingredients
½ zucchini, thinly sliced
½ red onion, thinly sliced
1 cup cherry tomatoes, halved
2 to 4 tablespoons pitted and chopped black olives
Pinch sea salt
Drizzle olive oil (optional)
2 prebaked pizza crusts
½ cup Classic Hummus**, or** Roasted Red Pepper Hummus
2 to 4 tablespoons **Cheesy Sprinkle**
Directions
1.Preheat the oven to 400°F.
2.Place the zucchini, onion, cherry tomatoes, and olives in a large bowl, sprinkle them with the sea salt, and toss them a bit. Drizzle with a bit of olive oil (if using), to seal in the flavor and keep them from drying out in the oven.
3.Lay the two crusts out on a large baking sheet. Spread half the hummus on each crust, and top with the veggie mixture and some Cheesy Sprinkle.
4.Pop the pizzas in the oven for 20 to 30 minutes, or until the veggies are soft.
Make Ahead: For a shortcut, lightly sauté the veggies before putting them on the pizza, so you only have to bake it for a few minutes until warmed through. You could even use some leftover sautéed vegetables.

Maple Dijon Burgers

Total time: 50 minutes
Ingredients
1 red bell pepper
1 (19-ounce) can chickpeas, rinsed and drained, or 2 cups cooked
1 cup ground almonds
2 teaspoons Dijon mustard
2 teaspoons maple syrup
1 garlic clove, pressed
Juice of ½ lemon
1 teaspoon dried oregano
½ teaspoon dried sage
1 cup spinach
1 to 1½ cups rolled oats
Directions
1.Preheat the oven to 350°F. Line a large baking sheet with parchment paper.
2.Cut the red pepper in half, remove the stem and seeds, and put on the baking sheet cut side up in the oven. Roast in the oven while you prep the other ingredients.
3.Put the chickpeas in the food processor, along with the almonds, mustard, maple syrup, garlic, lemon juice, oregano, sage, and spinach. Pulse until things are thoroughly combined but not puréed. When the red pepper is softened a bit, about 10 minutes, add it to the processor along with the oats and pulse until they are chopped just enough to form patties.
4.If you don't have a food processor, mash the chickpeas with a potato masher or fork, and make sure everything else is chopped up as finely as possible, then stir together.
5.Scoop up ¼-cup portions and form into 12 patties, and lay them out on the baking sheet.
6.Put the burgers in the oven and bake until the outside is lightly browned, about 30 minutes.

Cajun Burgers

Total time: 55 minutes
Ingredients
FOR THE DRESSING
1 tablespoon tahini
1 tablespoon apple cider vinegar
2 teaspoons Dijon mustard
1 to 2 tablespoons water
1 to 2 garlic cloves, pressed
1 teaspoon dried basil
1 teaspoon dried thyme
½ teaspoon dried oregano
½ teaspoon dried sage
½ teaspoon smoked paprika
¼ teaspoon cayenne pepper
¼ teaspoon sea salt
Pinch freshly ground black pepper
FOR THE BURGERS
2 cups water
1 cup kasha (toasted buckwheat)
Pinch sea salt
2 carrots, grated
Handful fresh parsley, chopped
1 teaspoon olive oil (optional)
Directions for the dressing
1.In a medium bowl, whisk together the tahini, vinegar, and mustard until the mixture is very thick. Add 1 to 2 tablespoons water to thin it out, and whisk again until smooth.
2.Stir in the rest of the ingredients. Set aside for the flavors to blend.
Directions for the burgers
1.Put the water, buckwheat, and sea salt in a medium pot. Bring to a boil and let boil for 2 to 3 minutes, then turn down to low, cover, and simmer for 15 minutes. Buckwheat is fully cooked when it is soft and no liquid is left at the bottom of the pot. Do not stir the buckwheat while it is cooking.
2.Once the buckwheat is cooked, transfer it to a large bowl. Stir the grated carrot, fresh parsley, and all the dressing into the buckwheat. Scoop up ¼-cup portions and form into patties.
3.You can either panfry or bake the burgers. To panfry, heat a large skillet to medium, add 1 teaspoon olive oil, and cook the burgers about 5 minutes on the first side. Flip, and cook another 5 minutes. To bake them, put them on a baking sheet lined with parchment paper and bake at 350°F for about 30 minutes.

Grilled Seitan in Barbeque Sauce

Total time: 10 minutes
Ingredients
8 oz of seitan (thinly sliced or chopped in 1" chunks)
½ cup of barbecue sauce
Cubed vegetable of your choice (blanch)
Directions
To start, make sure to soak the skewers in the water to prevent burning.
Put seitan in a plastic bag or cover well with barbecue sauce in a
deep pan. Mix and allow marinating for at least an hour; much better if longer.
Heat a grill to medium-high temperature.
Meanwhile, thread the seitan and vegetables on the skewers alternately. Grill the skewers on both sides until the seitan is cooked and golden brown on both sides while brushing with barbecue sauce.
Dish with the food and serve.

Tofu Wraps Curried

Total time: 25 minutes
Ingredients
½ cup garden greens of your choice (shredded)
3 tbsp of mint sauce
4 tbsp of yogurt (non- dairy, heaped)
3 pcs of 200g of tofu (cut in 15 cubes)
2 tbsp of tandoori curry paste
2 tbsp of oil
2 large cloves of garlic (sliced)
2 small size of onions (sliced)
8 chapatis (whole-wheat)
2 pcs of limes (cut into quarters)
Directions
In a medium bowl, combine the garden greens, mint sauce and yogurt, and set aside.
In a medium bowl, mix the tofu, tandoori paste, and oil.
Heat a skillet over medium temperature and cook the tofu until cooked within. Stir in the garlic, onions, and cook for 3 more minutes. Turn the heat off.
Toast the chapatis in a preheated grill pan until golden brown and lay on a flat surface.
Spoon in the garden green mixture, top with the tofu mix, wrap, and serve warm.

Tempeh Quesadillas

Total time: 15 minutes
Ingredients
For marinating
8 oz tempeh (pasteurized and chopped)
1 tbsp of tamari sauce
1 tsp of pure maple syrup
½ tsp of ginger (grated)
1 tbsp of chipotle avocado
½ clove of garlic
For assembling
2 tbsp of grape seed oil (divided)
4 tbsp of cashew cheese (divided)
2 corn or tortilla (whole wheat)
2 tbsp of shallot (minced, divided)

Directions
In a medium bowl, mix all the marinating ingredients and allow the tempeh to sit for 30 minutes.
Heat some olive oil in a medium skillet and cook the tempeh on all sides until golden brown, 10 minutes.
Transfer to a plate and set aside.
Working in batches, heat some oil in a medium skillet and lay in a tortilla.
Spread some cashew cheese on top and add the shallots and tempeh. Cover with the other tortilla.
Cook until the bottom part of the tortilla is golden brown, then carefully flip and cook the other side until golden brown, 10 minutes.
Transfer to a plate, slice into 4 pieces and serve warm.

Baked Squash topped with Beans

Total time: 30 minutes

Ingredients

2 tbsp of oil
6 cloves of garlic (minced)
2 small size onion (diced)
2 small size of mild chili (diced finely)
700 g of butternut squash (cut into 1cm diced)
Salt and pepper to taste
2 tsp of paprika (smoked)
½ tsp of hot chili powder
½ tsp of cumin (ground)
½ tsp of coriander (ground)
800g of chopped tomatoes
800g of black beans (rinsed, drained)
50g of cheddar cheese (vegan, grated)

Directions

In a large frying pan, heat the oil and add the garlic, onion, chili, squash and pepper. Season well and cook for 5-10 minutes over medium heat until the onion is quite tender.
Add the spices, chopped tomatoes and black beans, and combine gently.
Cover with a lid, heat for another 5-10 minutes until the butternut squash is thoroughly cooked.
Place the grated cheese on top and allow melting.
Serve warm.

Mexican Lentil Soup

Total time: 55 minutes

Ingredients

2 tbsp of olive oil (extra virgin)
2 carrots (peeled, diced)
1 yellow onion (diced)
1 red bell pepper (diced)
2 celery stalks (diced)
1 tbsp of cumin
3 cloves of garlic (minced)
2 cups of green lentils (rinsed, picked over)
2 cups of tomatoes (diced) and the juice
8 cups of vegetable broth
½ tsp of salt
2 cans of green chile (diced)
¼ tsp of smoked paprika
1 tsp of oregano
1 avocado (peeled, pitted, diced and for garnish)
Cilantro (fresh, for garnish)
Hot sauce (optional and for serving)

Directions

In a large pot, heat the olive oil over medium heat and cook in the carrots, onion, bell pepper and celery until soften, 5 minutes. Season with the cumin, garlic, pepper and cook for another minute.
Mix in the lentils, tomatoes, broth, salt and green chilies. Bring to a boil, cover the lid, and simmer until the lentils soften, 10 to 15 minutes.
Adjust the taste with salt, black pepper, and dish the soup.
Top with the avocado, cilantro and hot sauce.

Black Bean and Quinoa Balls

Total time: 60 minutes
Ingredients
For black beans and quinoa balls
½ cup of quinoa
1 can of beans (black)
¼ cup of seeds (sesame)
½ tbsp of Sriracha
¼ cup of flour (oat) / bread crumbs
2 tbsp of tomato paste
2 tbsp of nutritional yeast
1 tsp of garlic (powder)
1/2 tbsp of fresh herbs (oregano or basil)
For sun- dried tomato sauce
½ cup of cherry tomatoes (halved)
½ cup of tomatoes (sun-dried)
1 tbsp apple cider vinegar (ACV)
1 clove garlic
2 tbsp of pine nuts (toasted)
2 tbsp of nutritional yeast
fresh basil
1 tsp of oregano
Salt and pepper to taste
For serving
½ cup of cherry tomatoes (halved)
Fresh basil

Directions

Quinoa balls and black beans
In a dish, add quinoa and a cup of water, and boil until softens and the water absorbs, 15 minutes. Fluff and allow cooling.
Meanwhile, mash the black beans in a medium bowl using a fork and mix in the sesame seeds, Sriracha, quinoa, crumbs of bread or oat flour, tomato paste, spices and nutritional yeast and combine together until even dough forms.
Dig up about 2 tbsp of dough and roll into balls (approximately 22-25 total). Line a baking sheet with parchment paper and arrange the balls on top.
Cook in the oven for at 380 F until golden brown, 35 to 40 minutes.
For the sun- dried tomato sauce
Put all the sauce ingredients in a food processor or blender and process until creamy texture forms.
Serve the quinoa and black beans balls with the sauce and whole-wheat sauce.

Teriyaki Tempeh Tacos

Total time: 40 minutes
Ingredients
Teriyaki Tacos
1 batch of tempeh
6 pcs of taco shells (gluten free)
Asian Slaw
1 cup of cabbage (green, shredded)
1 cup of cabbage (red, shredded)
1 cup of carrots (grated)
3 of scallions (chopped)
Dressing
¼ cup of apple cider vinegar (ACV)
2 tbsp of olive oil (extra virgin)
1 tbsp of lime juice
½ tbsp of tamari sauce
1 tbsp of pure maple syrup
1 tbsp of mustard (Dijon)
1 tbsp of sriracha or hot sauce
¼ tsp of salt and pepper to taste
Directions
Heat the olive oil in a medium skillet over medium heat and fry the tempeh in batches on both sides until golden brown, 10 minutes. Set aside.
In a medium bowl, mix all the ingredients for the Asian slaw and set aside.
In another bowl, mix the dressing's ingredients.
On each taco shell, divide the tempeh, slaw, and dressing.
Serve immediately.

Green Pea Fritters

Total time: 40 minutes
Ingredients
Fritters
2 cups of fresh canned peas
1 tbsp of olive oil (divided)
3 cloves of garlic (minced)
1 large size of white onion (diced)
1 tsp of soda (bicarbonate)
2 tbsp herbs (dried, chopped finely)
1 ½ cups of chickpea flour
Salt and pepper to taste
Herby yoghurt dipping sauce
1 cup of yoghurt (soy)
herbs (dried, chopped finely)
1 lemon (squeezed)

Directions
Set the oven to 350 F and use a baking paper to line a baking sheet.
In heated olive oil, sauté the garlic and onion until softened.
In a medium bowl, mash and mix the peas with the garlic and onion mixture, bicarbonate soda, herbs, chickpeas, salt and pepper until coarsely smooth mixture forms. Wet your hands and form 2-inch patties from the mixture and arrange on the baking tray.
Bake in the oven until golden brown and compacted.
Serve with the dipping sauce.
Dipping sauce
In a medium bowl, mix all the sauce's ingredients and serve immediately with the fritters.

Hearty Black Lentil Curry

Total time: 6 hours 35 minutes
Ingredients
1 cup of black lentils, rinsed and soaked overnight
14 ounce of chopped tomatoes
2 large white onions, peeled and sliced
1 1/2 teaspoon of minced garlic
1 teaspoon of grated ginger
1 red chili
1 teaspoon of salt
1/4 teaspoon of red chili powder
1 teaspoon of paprika
1 teaspoon of ground turmeric
2 teaspoons of ground cumin
2 teaspoons of ground coriander
1/2 cup of chopped coriander
4-ounce of vegetarian butter
4 fluid of ounce water
2 fluid of ounce vegetarian double cream

Directions:
Place a large pan over an average heat, add butter and let heat until melt.
Add the onion along with garlic and ginger and let cook for 10 to 15 minutes or until onions are caramelized.
Then stir in salt, red chili powder, paprika, turmeric, cumin, ground coriander, and water.
Transfer this mixture to a 6-quarts slow cooker and add tomatoes and red chili.
Drain lentils, add to slow cooker and stir until just mix.
Plug in slow cooker; adjust cooking time to 6 hours and let cook on low heat setting.
When the lentils are done, stir in cream and adjust the seasoning.
Serve with boiled rice or whole wheat bread.

Flavorful Refried Beans

Total time: 8 hours 15 minutes
Ingredients
3 cups of pinto beans, rinsed
1 small jalapeno pepper, seeded and chopped
1 medium-sized white onion, peeled and sliced
2 tablespoons of minced garlic
5 teaspoons of salt
2 teaspoons of ground black pepper
1/4 teaspoon of ground cumin
9 cups of water

Directions:
Using a 6-quarts slow cooker, place all the ingredients and stir until it mixes properly.
Cover the top, plug in the slow cooker; adjust the cooking time to 6 hours, let it cook on high heat setting and add more water if the beans get too dry.
When the beans are done, drain them and reserve the liquid.
Mash the beans using a potato masher and pour in the reserved cooking liquid until it reaches your desired mixture.
Serve immediately.

Chunky Black Lentil Veggie Soup

Total time: 4 hours 35 minutes
Ingredients
1 1/2 cups of black lentils, uncooked
2 small turnips, peeled and diced
10 medium-sized carrots, peeled and diced
1 medium-sized green bell pepper, cored and diced
3 cups of diced tomatoes
1 medium-sized white onion, peeled and diced
2 tablespoons of minced ginger
1 teaspoon of minced garlic
1 teaspoon of salt
1/2 teaspoon of ground coriander
1/2 teaspoon of ground cumin
3 tablespoons of unsalted butter
32 fluid ounce of vegetable broth
32 fluid ounce of water
Directions:
Using a medium-sized microwave, cover the bowl, place the lentils and pour in the water.
Microwave lentils for 10 minutes or until softened, stirring after 5 minutes.
Drain lentils and add to a 6-quarts slow cooker along with remaining ingredients and stir until just mix.
Cover with top, plug in slow cooker; adjust cooking time to 6 hours and let cook on low heat setting or until carrots are tender.
Serve straight away.

Exotic Butternut Squash and Chickpea Curry

Total time: 6 hours 15 minutes
Ingredients
1 1/2 cups of shelled peas
1 1/2 cups of chick peas, uncooked and rinsed
2 1/2 cups of diced butternut squash
12 ounce of chopped spinach
2 large tomatoes, diced
1 small white onion, peeled and chopped
1 teaspoon of minced garlic
1 teaspoon of salt
3 tablespoons of curry powder
14-ounce of coconut milk
3 cups of vegetable broth
1/4 cup of chopped cilantro
Directions:
Using a 6-quarts slow cooker, place all the ingredients into it except for the spinach and peas.
Cover the top, plug in the slow cooker; adjust the cooking time to 6 hours and let it cook on the high heat setting or until the chickpeas get tender.
30 minutes to ending your cooking, add the peas and spinach to the slow cooker and let it cook for the remaining 30 minutes.
Stir to check the sauce, if the sauce is runny, stir in a mixture of a tablespoon of cornstarch mixed with 2 tablespoons of water.
Serve with boiled rice.

Lovely Parsnip & Split Pea Soup

Total time: 5 hours 10 minutes
Ingredients
1 tablespoon of olive oil
2 large parsnips, peeled and chopped
2 large carrots, peeled and chopped
1 medium-sized white onion, peeled and diced
1 1/2 teaspoon of minced garlic
2 1/4 cups of dried green split peas, rinsed
1 teaspoon of salt
1/2 teaspoon of ground black pepper
1 teaspoon of dried thyme
2 bay leaves
6 cups of vegetable broth
1 teaspoon of liquid smoke
Directions:
Place a medium-sized non-stick skillet pan over an average pressure of heat, add the oil and let it heat.
Add the parsnip, carrot, onion, garlic and let it cook for 5 minutes or until it is heated.
Transfer this mixture into a 6-quarts slow cooker and add the remaining ingredients.
Stir until mixes properly and cover the top.
Plug in the slow cooker; adjust the cooking time to 5 hours and let it cook on the high heat setting or until the peas and vegetables get soft.
When done, remove the bay leaf from the soup and blend it with a submersion blender or until the soup reaches your desired state.
Add the seasoning and serve.

Incredible Tomato Basil Soup

Total time: 6 hours 10 minutes
Ingredients
1 cup of chopped celery
1 cup of chopped carrots
74 ounce of whole tomatoes, canned
2 cups of chopped white onion
2 teaspoons of minced garlic
1 tablespoon of salt
1/2 teaspoon of ground white pepper
1/4 cup of basil leaves and more for garnishing
1 bay leaf
32 fluid ounce of vegetable broth
1/2 cup of grated Parmesan cheese
Directions:
Using an 8 quarts or larger slow cooker, place all the ingredients.
Stir until it mixes properly and cover the top.
Plug in the slow cooker; adjust the cooking time to 5 hours and let it cook on the high heat setting or until the vegetables are tender.
Blend the soup with a submersion blender or until soup reaches your desired state.
Garnish it with the cheese, basil leaves and serve.

Sizzling Vegetarian Fajitas

Total time: 2 hours 25 minutes
Ingredients
4 ounce of diced green chilies
3 medium-sized tomatoes, diced
1 large green bell pepper, cored and sliced
1 large red bell pepper, cored and sliced
1 medium-sized white onion, peeled and sliced
1/2 teaspoon of garlic powder
1/4 teaspoon of salt
2 teaspoons of red chili powder
2 teaspoons of ground cumin
1/2 teaspoon of dried oregano
1 1/2 tablespoon of olive oil
Directions:
Take a 6-quarts slow cooker, grease it with a non-stick cooking spray and add all the ingredients.
Stir until it mixes properly and cover the top.
Plug in the slow cooker; adjust the cooking time to 2 hours and let it cook on the high heat setting or until cooks thoroughly.
Serve with tortillas.

Rich Red Lentil Curry

Total time: 8 hours 10 minutes
Ingredients
4 cups of brown lentils, uncooked and rinsed
2 medium-sized white onions, peeled and diced
2 teaspoons of minced garlic
1 tablespoon of minced ginger
1 teaspoon of salt
1/4 teaspoon of cayenne pepper
5 tablespoons of red curry paste
2 teaspoon of brown sugar
1 1/2 teaspoon of ground turmeric
1 tablespoon of garam masala
60-ounce of tomato puree
7 cups of water
1/2 cup of coconut milk
1/4 cup of chopped cilantro
Directions:
Using a 6-quarts slow cooker, place all the ingredients except for the coconut milk and cilantro.
Stir until it mixes properly and cover the top.
Plug in the slow cooker; adjust the cooking time to 5 hours and let it cook on the high heat setting or until the lentils are soft.
Check the curry during cooking and add more water if needed.
When the curry is cooked, stir in the milk, then garnish it with the cilantro and serve right away.

Smoky Red Beans and Rice

Total time: 5 hours 10 minutes
Ingredients
30 ounce of cooked red beans
1 cup of brown rice, uncooked
1 cup of chopped green pepper
1 cup of chopped celery
1 cup of chopped white onion
1 1/2 teaspoon of minced garlic
1/2 teaspoon of salt
1/4 teaspoon of cayenne pepper
1 teaspoon of smoked paprika
2 teaspoons of dried thyme
1 bay leaf
2 1/3 cups of vegetable broth
Directions:
Using a 6-quarts slow cooker place all the ingredients except for the rice, salt and cayenne pepper.
Stir until it mixes properly and then cover the top.
Plug in the slow cooker; adjust the cooking time to 4 hours and let it steam on a low heat setting.
Then pour in and stir the rice, salt, cayenne pepper and continue cooking for an additional 2 hours at a high heat setting.
Serve straight away.

Spicy Black-Eyed Peas

Total time: 8 hours 20 minutes
Ingredients
32-ounce black-eyed peas, uncooked
1 cup of chopped orange bell pepper
1 cup of chopped celery
8-ounce of chipotle peppers, chopped
1 cup of chopped carrot
1 cup of chopped white onion
1 teaspoon of minced garlic
3/4 teaspoon of salt
1/2 teaspoon of ground black pepper
2 teaspoons of liquid smoke flavoring
2 teaspoons of ground cumin
1 tablespoon of adobo sauce
2 tablespoons of olive oil
1 tablespoon of apple cider vinegar
4 cups of vegetable broth
Directions:
Place a medium-sized non-stick skillet pan over an average temperature of heat; add the bell peppers, carrot, onion, garlic, oil and vinegar.
Stir until it mixes properly and let it cook for 5 to 8 minutes or until it gets translucent.
Transfer this mixture to a 6-quarts slow cooker and add the peas, chipotle pepper, adobo sauce and the vegetable broth.
Stir until mixes properly and cover the top.
Plug in the slow cooker; adjust the cooking time to 8 hours and let it cook on the low heat setting or until peas are soft.
Serve right away.

Vegan Spinach Ricotta Lasagna

Total time: 75 minutes

Ingredients

Cashew ricotta cheese
2 cups of cashews (raw)
¾ cups of water
1 lemon (squeezed)
2 cloves of garlic (grated)
½ tsp onion (powder)
½ tsp of garlic (powder)
½ tsp of sea salt
Lasagna
½ onion (diced)
1 lb mushrooms (sliced)
6 cups of baby spinach
4 ½ cups of tomato sauce
12 oz of lasagna noodles (no boil lentil)
6 oz of vegan smoked Gouda cheese slices
1 large heirloom tomato (sliced)
1/3 cup of basil leaves (garnish)
A pinch of red pepper (flakes)

Directions

Cashew Ricotta

Wash the cashews thoroughly for 20 minutes, drain and blend in a food processor until smooth. Set aside in the refrigerator until needed.

Preparing the oven

In a large saucepan, steam the onion with a teaspoon of water. Add the mushrooms and simmer for 10 minutes. Season with salt to taste.

Pour another teaspoon of water in the same pan and cook in the spinach until wilted. Drain and set aside.

Spread 1 ½ cups of tomato sauce in a medium baking pan and lay in half of the noodles.

Spread a third of the ricotta cashew on top, add a third of the spinach mixture and repeat the layering process two more times making sure to top finally with the ricotta cashew cheese.

Layer the vegan smoked gouda layer on top and the sliced tomatoes on top.

Cover with foil and bake in the oven for 45 to 60 minutes or until the cheeses melt.

Remove from the oven, allow cooling for 5 minutes, top with the basil, slice and serve.

Spice- crusted Tofu with Kumquat Radish Salad

Total time: 5 minutes
Ingredients
200g of tofu (firm)
2 tbsp of sesame seeds
1 tbsp spice mix (Japanese shichimi togarashi)
½ tbsp of cornflour
1 tbsp of vegetable oil
200g of broccoli (Tender stem)
100g of sugar
5 radishes (sliced)
2 spring onions (chopped)
2 kumquats (sliced)
1 tbsp of sesame oil
For the dressing
2 tbsp of tamari sauce
2 tbsp of lime juice
1 tsp of golden caster sugar
1 small shallot (diced finely)
1 tsp of ginger (grated)
Directions
Cut the tofu in two and press with parchment paper. Cut into chunky slices.
In a cup, mix the sesame seeds, Also mix the Japanese spice mix and corn flour. Slather the mixture and get it covered.
Heat the olive oil in a large skillet and fry the tofu on both sides, 10 minutes. Set aside in a large salad bowl.
Steam the broccoli and snap peas in a microwave until softened, 2 to 3 minutes.
In the salad bowl, add the broccoli, snap peas, radishes, spring onion and kumquats.
Mix the dressing's ingredients in a medium bowl and serve with the salad.

Mongolian Seitan

Total time: 30 minutes
Ingredients
For seitan
1 ½ tbsp of vegetable oil
1 lb of seitan (cut into 1-inch pcs)
For the Mongolian sauce
2 tsp of oil (vegetable)
3 cloves of garlic (minced)
1/2 tsp of ginger (minced)
1/3 tsp of five spice (optional)
1/3 tsp of red pepper (flakes)
1/2 cup of tamari sauce
1/2 cup + 2 tbsp sugar (coconut)
2 tbsp of cold water
2 tsp of cornstarch
For serving
sesame seeds (toasted, optional)
scallions (sliced, optional)
Directions
For the seitan
Heat the vegetable oil in a saucepan in a medium - high heat and cook in the seitan until golden brown on both sides, 10 minutes.
For the sauce:
Meanwhile, as the seitan cooks, warm the vegetable oil over medium heat in a pan.
Sauté the garlic, ginger, five spice (optional) and red pepper flakes until fragrant, 30 seconds.
Mix in the tamari sauce, coconut sugar and cook over low heat until the sugar melts.
In a small bowl, mix the cornstarch and cold water, and mix into the sauce. Cook for 1 minute.
Mix in the seitan, cook for 1 minute, and top with the sesame seeds and scallions.
Dish the food and serve warm.

Red Lentil Quinoa Fritters

Total time: 45 minutes
Ingredients
Red lentil quinoa fritters
½ *cup of* red lentils
1 ½ cup of quinoa
4 cups of water
2 tsp of turmeric (ground)
½ lemon (squeezed)
1 tsp of cumin
½ tsp of salt and pepper to taste
¼ tsp of cinnamon (ground)
¼ *cup of* chickpea flour
¼ cup or cornmeal
¼ cup of fresh parsley (chopped)
¼ cup of tahini
1 tbsp of mustard (Dijon)
Tahini yogurt sauce
1 cup plant-based yogurt
3 tbsp tahini
juice of 1 lemon
2 minced garlic cloves
1 tbsp chopped fresh dill
1/4 tsp salt (or to taste)

Directions
For the fritters:
Set the oven for 400F and line a baking tray with parchment paper.
Wash and flush the lentils and quinoa. In a medium saucepan, boil lentils and quinoa for 15 minutes. Mix/stir well intermediary to avoid burning. Reserve to cool.
In a large mixing container, mix the turmeric, lemon juice, cumin, salt, and cinnamon until well combined.
Incorporate the chickpea flour and cornmeal into the mixture until moist dough forms. Mold 1-inch patties from the mixture and arrange on the baking tray.
Bake in the oven for 15 minutes while flipping halfway until the patties are golden brown and well compacted. Serve with the tahini yogurt sauce.
For the tahini yogurt sauce:
While still cooking the fritters, combine all the ingredients for the tahini yogurt sauce. Reserve until serving time.

Easy Vegan Chili Sin Carne

Total time: 30 minutes
Ingredients
2 tbsp of olive oil
1 large size of red onion (slice thinly)
3 cloves of garlic (minced)
2 medium size carrots (peeled, chopped finely)
2 small size red pepper (chopped roughly)
2 celery stalks (chopped finely)
1 tsp of chili powder
Salt and pepper to taste
1 tsp of cumin (ground)
400g of red kidney beans (rinsed and drained)
800g of chopped tomatoes (tinned)
100g of red lentils (split)
250ml of vegetable stock
400g of soy mince (frozen)
Directions
Heat the olive oil in a large saucepan over medium heat.
Cook in the onion, garlic, carrots, pepper and celery until softened, 5 minutes.
Mix in the chili powder, salt, pepper, and cumin powder.
Add the kidney beans, tomatoes, lentils, vegetable stock and thin soy. Cook for 15 minutes and adjust the taste with salt and black pepper.
Dish the food and serve with cooked quinoa.

Fall Farro Protein Bowl

Total time: 45 minutes
Ingredients
1 cup of carrots (1/2 inch diced)
1 cup of sweet potato (1/2 inch diced)
2 tsp of organic oil (divided)
Salt and pepper to taste (divided)
15oz of chickpeas (rinsed and drained)
4oz of smoky tempeh strips
½ cup of farro (uncooked)
1 ¼ cups of water
2 cups of mixed greens
¼ cup of hummus
2 tbsp of roasted almonds
4 slices of lemon (wedges)
Directions
Heat the oven to 375 F and prepare a large baking tray.
In a large mixing bowl, mix the carrots and sweet potatoes with 1 tsp of cooking oil and a pinch of salt and pepper. Spread the mixture on the baking sheet.
In the same mixing container, place the chickpeas and a tsp of oil, a pinch of salt and 1/8 tsp of pepper, and mix well.
Spread the mixture on the vegetables and top with the tempeh strips.
Bake in the oven for until the sweet potatoes are tender, 30 minutes. Remove the food from the oven and set aside.
Meanwhile as the vegetables baked, cook the farro in a slightly salted water in a medium pot over medium heat until softened and the water absorbs, 10 to 15 minutes.
To serve, divide the farro and mixed greens between four bowls. Share the tempeh mixture likewise as well as the other ingredients.
Serve warm.

Stir- fried Sprout with Green Beans, Lemon and Pine Nuts

Total time: 10 minutes

Ingredients

300g of Brussels sprouts (trimmed, cut in quarter)
300g of green beans
1 tbsp of olive oil
1 small lemon (zest and squeezed)
2 tbsp of pine nuts (toasted)

Directions

In a pan of boiling salted water, cook the sprouts and beans for 3 minutes, then drain well afterwards.
Heat the olive oil in a medium skillet over medium heat and stir-fry the vegetables.
Mix in the lemon zest, lemon juice, and pine nuts. Cook for 3 minutes and turn the heat off.
Dish the food and serve warm.

Potato Tofu Quiche

Total time: 90 minutes

Ingredients

For the crust
1 ½ medium size potatoes (grated)
1 tbsp of sea salt and pepper
1 tbsp of melted vegan butter
For the filling
½ cup of chopped broccoli
1 ½ cloves of garlic (chopped)
1 medium size of leeks (sliced thinly)
1 tbsp melted vegan butter
1 tbsp of nutritional yeast
Sea salt and pepper to taste
1 ½ tbsp of hummus
6 oz of tofu (extra- firm silken, dried)
3 cups of cherry tomatoes (halves)

Directions

Set the oven to 450 degrees F and gently dab a 9.5-inch baking pan with non-stick spray.
Spread the potatoes on the baking sheet and season with the salt, pepper, and butter.
In another baking sheet, mix the broccoli, garlic, leeks, and season with salt, black pepper, and drizzle the vegan butter on top.
Place both sheets in the oven and bake until the vegetables are tender and golden brown, 25 to 30 minutes.
Transfer the vegetables to a food processor and top with the remaining ingredients. Process until coarsely combined.
Pour the mixture into a pre-greased loaf pan and bake in the oven until golden brown and compacted, 30 to 40 minutes.
Remove the pan from the oven, allow cooling for 3 minutes and invert the quiche onto a flat surface.
Slice and serve.

Black bean and Seitan Stir- fry

Total time: 25 minutes
Ingredients
400g of black beans (drained, rinsed)
75g of pure date sugar
3 cloves of garlic
2 tbsp of tamari sauce
1 tsp of five- spice (powder)
2 tbsp of wine vinegar
1 tbsp of peanut butter (smooth)
1 small size red chili (chopped finely)
350g of marinated seitan (piece)
1 small size shallots (chopped)
1 tbsp of corn flour
2 to 3 tbsp of vegetable oil
1 small size red bell pepper (sliced)
2 small size spring onions (sliced)
300g of pak choi (chopped)
Directions
Begin by preparing the sauce. In a food processor, add the black beans, date sugar, garlic, tamari sauce, five-spice powder, wine vinegar, peanut butter, and red chili. Process until smooth and pour the mixture into a medium pot. Heat the mixture over medium heat until thickened, 5 minutes.
Wash and drain the seitan using a paper towel. Add the seitan in a container together with the corn flour and reserve for later. Warm your saucepan to a high temperature, heat in some oil and fry the seitan until golden brown on both sides, 10 minutes. Transfer to a plate and set aside.
Heat a teaspoon of oil in the pot and sauté the shallots, peppers, spring onion, and pak choi until softened, 3 minutes.
Mix in the seitan, top with the sauce, toss well, and serve immediately.

Chapter 7: Dinner Recipes

Sweet Potato Patties

Total time: 35 minutes

Ingredients

1 cup cooked short-grain brown rice, fully cooled
1 cup grated sweet potato
½ cup diced onion
Pinch sea salt
¼ cup fresh parsley, finely chopped
1 tablespoon dried dill, or 2 tablespoons fresh
1 to 2 tablespoons nutritional yeast (optional)
½ cup whole-grain flour, or bread crumbs, or gluten-free flour
1 teaspoon olive oil

Directions

1.Stir together the rice, sweet potato, onion, and salt in a large bowl. Allow it to sit for a few minutes, so that the salt can draw the moisture out of the potato and onion. Stir in the parsley, dill, and nutritional yeast (if using), then add enough flour to make the batter sticky, adding a spoonful or two of water if necessary.
2.Form the mixture into tight balls, and squish slightly into patties.
3.Heat a large skillet on medium, then add the oil. Cook for 7 to 10 minutes, then flip. Cook another 5 to 7 minutes, and serve.

Make ahead: Be sure your rice is thoroughly cooled before you begin, or it will not be sticky enough to make into a patty. This is a great way to use up leftover rice.

Simple Sesame Stir-Fry

Total time: 30 minutes

Ingredients

1 cup quinoa
2 cups water
Pinch sea salt
1 head broccoli
1 to 2 teaspoons untoasted sesame oil, or olive oil
1 cup snow peas, or snap peas, ends trimmed and cut in half
1 cup frozen shelled edamame beans, or peas
2 cups chopped Swiss chard, or other large-leafed green
2 scallions, chopped
2 tablespoons water
1 teaspoon toasted sesame oil
1 tablespoon tamari, or soy sauce
2 tablespoons sesame seeds

Directions

1.Put the quinoa, water, and sea salt in a medium pot, bring it to a boil for a minute, then turn to low and simmer, covered, for 20 minutes. The quinoa is fully cooked when you see the swirl of the grains with a translucent center, and it is fluffy. Do not stir the quinoa while it is cooking.
2.Meanwhile, cut the broccoli into bite-size florets, cutting and pulling apart from the stem. Also chop the stem into bite-size pieces.
3.Heat a large skillet to high, and sauté the broccoli in the untoasted sesame oil, with a pinch of salt to help it soften. Keep this moving continuously, so that it doesn't burn, and add an extra drizzle of oil if needed as you add the rest of the vegetables. Add the snow peas next, continuing to stir. Add the edamame until they thaw. Add the Swiss chard and scallions at the same time, tossing for only a minute to wilt. Then add 2 tablespoons of water to the hot skillet so that it sizzles and finishes the vegetables with a quick steam.
4.Dress with the toasted sesame oil and tamari, and toss one last time. Remove from the heat immediately.
5.Serve a scoop of cooked quinoa, topped with stir-fry and sprinkled with some sesame seeds, and an extra drizzle of tamari and/or toasted sesame oil if you like.

Options: I went for a green theme here, but make this with pretty much any vegetables you like (or have left in the fridge): bell peppers, carrots, mushrooms, eggplant, zucchini, cherry tomatoes. Just think through which take the longest to cook, and add them first, finishing with whatever takes the least time to cook.

Spaghetti and Buckwheat Meatballs

Total time: 65 minutes
Ingredients
FOR THE BUCKWHEAT MEATBALLS
½ cup toasted buckwheat
2¼ cups water, divided
Pinch sea salt
2 tablespoons ground flaxseed, or chia seeds
2 tablespoons tomato paste, or ketchup
1 tablespoon stone-ground mustard
2 tablespoons tamari, or soy sauce
1 tablespoon mixed dried herbs (basil, oregano, marjoram)
1 teaspoon onion powder
1 teaspoon garlic powder
½ teaspoon ground cumin
½ teaspoon smoked paprika, or regular paprika
FOR THE SPAGHETTI
7 ounces whole-grain spaghetti, or ½ spaghetti squash
2 cups Marinara Sauce
2 to 3 tablespoons **Cheesy Sprinkle**

Directions
1.Preheat the oven to 350°F. Lightly grease a large rectangular baking sheet with olive oil, or line it with parchment paper.
2.Put the buckwheat in a small pot with 2 cups of the water and the salt, and bring to a boil. Turn the heat down and simmer, covered, for about 5 minutes. (If you use untoasted buckwheat, it will take closer to 20 minutes to cook after boiling.)
3.In a small bowl, mix the ground flaxseed with the remaining ¼ cup water and set aside.
4.In a large bowl, mix the tomato paste, mustard, tamari, herbs, onion powder, garlic powder, cumin, and paprika. Add the cooked buckwheat and soaked flax and stir to combine.
5.Shape spoonfuls of the mix into 20 to 24 small balls. Transfer to the baking sheet and put in the oven for 30 minutes.
6.Cook the spaghetti (or spaghetti squash) by putting it in a pot of boiling water and boiling until soft, about 10 minutes (15 to 20 for the squash). Drain the pasta, or scoop the flesh out of the squash's skin.
7.Once the meatballs are done, take them out of the oven and let cool for a few minutes.
8.Serve a plate of spaghetti (or squash) topped with Marinara Sauce, a few buckwheat meatballs, and Cheesy Sprinkle.

Orange Walnut Pasta

Total time: 40 minutes
Ingredients
½ spaghetti squash, or 7 ounces whole-grain pasta, or 14 ounces mixed vegetables
Zest and juice of 1 orange
2 tablespoons olive oil
1 garlic clove, pressed
Pinch sea salt
2 to 3 tablespoons fresh parsley, finely chopped
10 olives, pitted and chopped
¼ cup walnuts, chopped
2 to 3 tablespoons nutritional yeast (optional)
1.Cook your noodle of choice:
Directions
•Spaghetti squash: Boil until soft, about 15 to 20 minutes. Scoop the flesh out of the skin. Drain for a few minutes.
•Whole-grain pasta: Put it in a pot of boiling water with a pinch salt and cook until just soft, about 10 to 15 minutes. Drain.
•Mixed vegetables: Peel, and cut the ends flat to each other. Run through a spiralizer, or use a vegetable peeler to make long noodles. Either have them raw (in which case, you can toss with a sprinkle of salt and leave to soften and drain for 20 to 30 minutes), or cook lightly by steaming or boiling for just a few minutes.
2.In a large bowl, add the orange zest and juice. Whisk in an amount of olive oil that's about half the volume of the orange juice, along with the pressed garlic, and the salt; stir to blend. Add the noodles to the dressing, and toss.
3.Serve topped with a sprinkling of fresh parsley, chopped olives, walnuts, and a dusting of nutritional yeast (if using).

Roasted Cauliflower Tacos

Total time: 40 minutes
Ingredients
FOR THE ROASTED CAULIFLOWER
1 head cauliflower, cut into bite-size pieces
1 tablespoon olive oil (optional)
2 tablespoons whole-grain flour
2 tablespoons nutritional yeast
1 to 2 teaspoons smoked paprika
½ to 1 teaspoon chili powder
Pinch sea salt
FOR THE TACOS
2 cups shredded lettuce
2 cups cherry tomatoes, quartered
2 carrots, scrubbed or peeled, and grated
½ cup Fresh Mango Salsa
½ cup **Guacamole**
8 small whole-grain or corn tortillas
1 lime, cut into 8 wedges
Directions
TO MAKE THE ROASTED CAULIFLOWER
1.Preheat the oven to 350°F. Lightly grease a large rectangular baking sheet with olive oil, or line it with parchment paper.
2.In a large bowl, toss the cauliflower pieces with oil (if using), or just rinse them so they're wet. The idea is to get the seasonings to stick.
3.In a smaller bowl, mix together the flour, nutritional yeast, paprika, chili powder, and salt. Add the seasonings to the cauliflower, and mix it around with your hands to thoroughly coat.
4.Spread the cauliflower on the baking sheet, and roast for 20 to 30 minutes, or until softened.
TO MAKE THE TACOS
1.Prep the veggies, salsa, and guacamole while the cauliflower is roasting.
2.Once the cauliflower is cooked, heat the tortillas for just a few minutes in the oven or in a small skillet.
3.Set everything out on the table, and assemble your tacos as you go. Give a squeeze of fresh lime just before eating.
Leftovers: Double the batch of roasted cauliflower and add it to salads, bowls, and wraps, or serve as a side dish with **Avo-nnaise**.

Build Your Own Mushroom Fajitas

Total time: 40 minutes
Ingredients
FOR THE SPICY GLAZED MUSHROOMS
1 (10- to 12-ounce) package cremini mushrooms
1 teaspoon olive oil
½ to 1 teaspoon chili powder
Pinch freshly ground black pepper
Pinch sea salt
1 teaspoon maple syrup
FOR THE FAJITAS
1 onion
1 to 2 teaspoons olive oil, or 1 tablespoon vegetable broth or water
Pinch sea salt
1 zucchini, cut into large matchsticks
1 bell pepper, any color, seeded and sliced into long strips
½ cup fresh cilantro, finely chopped
3 to 4 scallions, sliced
2 carrots, grated
6 whole-grain or corn tortilla wraps
Guacamole
Fresh Mango Salsa
Cashew Sour Cream
Your favorite hot sauce (optional)
Directions
TO MAKE THE SPICY GLAZED MUSHROOMS
1.To glaze the mushrooms, wipe them clean with a paper towel, then cut them into thin slices.
2.Heat the oil in a large skillet over medium heat, then sauté the mushrooms until soft, about 10 minutes. Add the chili powder, pepper, and salt and stir to coat the mushrooms. Add the maple syrup to the skillet, stir to coat, and allow to cook for a few minutes to create a glaze.
3.Transfer the mushrooms to a heatproof dish, and keep them warm in the oven on very low, or allow them to cool if you aren't particular.
TO MAKE THE FAJITAS
1.Cut the onion in half from stem to tip. Then slice the strips perpendicular to that cut, so they make half moons. Separate the layers into arclike shapes.
2.Rinse the mushroom skillet if you want to clear the flavors, or leave it as is, and put the skillet back on the heat. Sauté the onion in the olive oil and salt. Once the onion is translucent, about 5 minutes, add the zucchini and bell pepper, and sauté until they're soft, 7 to 8 minutes.
3.While the zucchini is cooking, prepare the cilantro, scallions, and carrots.
4.Heat your tortilla wraps for a few minutes in a toaster oven, oven, or dry skillet. Place everything on the table so each person can assemble their own fajita.

Sun-dried Tomato and Pesto Quinoa

Total time: 25 minutes
Ingredients
1 teaspoon olive oil, or 1 tablespoon vegetable broth or water
1 cup chopped onion
1 garlic clove, minced
1 cup chopped zucchini
Pinch sea salt
1 tomato, chopped
2 tablespoons chopped sun-dried tomatoes
2 to 3 tablespoons **Basil Pesto**
1 cup chopped spinach
2 cups cooked quinoa
1 tablespoon **Cheesy Sprinkle**, optional
Directions
1.Heat the oil in a large skillet on medium-high, then sauté the onion, about 5 minutes. Add the garlic when the onion has softened, then add the zucchini and salt.
2.Once the zucchini is somewhat soft, about 5 minutes, turn off the heat and add the fresh and sun-dried tomatoes. Mix to combine, then toss in the pesto. Toss the vegetables to coat them.
3.Layer the spinach, then quinoa, then the zucchini mixture on a plate, topped with a bit of Cheesy Sprinkle (if using).
Options: This is a great way to use leftover cooked quinoa, but this dish is also nice with whole-grain pasta.

Olive and White Bean Pasta

Total time: 30 minutes
Ingredients
½ cup whole-grain pasta
Pinch sea salt
1 teaspoon olive oil, or 1 tablespoon vegetable broth
¼ cup thinly sliced red bell pepper
¼ cup thinly sliced zucchini
½ cup cooked cannellini beans
½ cup spinach
1 tablespoon balsamic vinegar
2 or 3 black olives, pitted and chopped
1 tablespoon nutritional yeast
Directions
1.Bring a pot of water to a boil, then add the pasta with the salt to cook until just tender (per the package directions).
2.Meanwhile, in a large skillet, heat the oil and lightly sauté the bell pepper and zucchini, 7 to 8 minutes. Add the beans to warm for 2 minutes, then add the spinach last, just until it wilts. Drizzle with the vinegar at the end.
3.Serve the pasta topped or tossed with the bean mixture, and sprinkled with the olives and nutritional yeast.
Options: Use brown rice, quinoa, or corn pasta to easily make this dish gluten-free. It would also be nice with cooked basmati rice instead of pasta.

Vietnamese Summer Rolls

Total time: 60 minutes
Ingredients
10 round rice roll wraps
¼ cup fresh basil, mint, cilantro, or parsley leaves (or a combination)
10 palm-size lettuce leaves (either small leaves, or tear larger leaves into smaller pieces)
2 carrots, grated or julienned
½ cucumber, julienned
1 mango, peeled and sliced into long, thin pieces
3 scallions, sliced lengthwise into quarters
1 cup bean sprouts
½ cup Peanut Sauce
Directions
1.Fill a deep plate with room-temperature water, and put a rice roll wrap in to soften. It will take a couple of minutes to get very soft. Pull it out of the water and allow it to drip for a few seconds, then place it on a dry plate.
2.Down the center of the wrap, lay 2 fresh basil leaves and a lettuce leaf, then cover with the carrots, cucumber, mango, scallions, and bean sprouts. Don't overfill, or it will be difficult to roll.
3.Fold over the top and bottom of the rice wrap, then fold one side over the filling and tuck it under the filling a bit. Squeeze slightly with your hands and then roll to the end of the other side. Allow the wraps to sit and stick together before serving.
4.Slice each wrap in half, and serve with Peanut Sauce for dipping.
Technique: Put the next wrap in the water to soften while you roll the current one, so that you don't have to wait for them to soften each time.

Potato Skin Samosas

Total time: 50 minutes
Ingredients
4 small baking potatoes
1 teaspoon coconut oil
1 small onion, finely chopped
2 garlic cloves, minced
1 small piece ginger, minced or grated
2 to 3 teaspoons curry powder
Pinch sea salt
Pinch freshly ground black pepper
2 carrots, grated
¼ cup frozen peas, thawed
¼ cup fresh cilantro, or parsley, chopped
Directions
1.Preheat the oven to 350°F.
2.Pierce the potatoes with a fork, wrap them in aluminum foil, and bake 30 minutes, or until soft.
3.While the potatoes are cooking, heat the oil in a medium skillet and sauté the onion until it's soft, about 5 minutes. Add the garlic and ginger and sauté until they're soft as well, about 3 minutes. Add the curry powder, salt, and pepper, and stir to fully coat the onion. Turn off the heat.
4.When the potatoes are cooked, take them out of the foil and slice them in half.
6.If you like, you can prepare these in advance and then heat them up in the oven at 350°F for 10 minutes when you're ready to serve.
Toppings: Cashew Sour Cream is lovely with these, as is a drizzle of **Peanut Sauce**. Or you could try **Fresh Mango Salsa**.

Spicy Chickpea Sushi Rolls

Total time: 75 minutes
Ingredients
FOR THE SUSHI RICE
1 cup short-grain brown rice
2 cups water
Pinch sea salt
1 to 2 tablespoons brown rice vinegar
FOR THE SPICY CHICKPEA FILLING
½ cup cooked chickpeas
2 to 3 scallions, finely chopped
⅛ teaspoon cayenne pepper (more or less, to your taste)
1 to 2 tablespoons **Avo-nnaise**
FOR THE SUSHI ROLLS
3 cups cooked sushi rice
4 nori sheets
¼ cucumber, julienned
TO SERVE
Tamari or soy sauce
1 tablespoon pickled ginger
1 teaspoon wasabi
Directions
TO MAKE THE SUSHI RICE
1.Put the rice and water in a large pot. Add a bit of sea salt, bring to a boil for a couple of minutes, then turn to low and simmer, covered, for 45 minutes. The rice is fully cooked when it is dry and fluffy. Do not stir the rice while it is cooking. This will yield about 3 to 3½ cups sushi rice, which is the perfect amount for 4 rolls.
2.Transfer the rice to a large bowl so that it can fully cool. Stir in the vinegar, just enough to make the rice stick to itself, along with another sprinkle of salt. Stir the rice occasionally to speed up the cooling. You can also put it in the fridge to cool it more quickly.
TO MAKE THE SPICY CHICKPEA FILLING
Mash the chickpeas with a potato masher, fork, or your hands. Mix in the scallions, cayenne, and just enough Avo-nnaise to make it stick together. You don't want this to be too creamy, or it will make your sushi soggy.
TO MAKE THE SUSHI ROLLS
1.Set out a small dish of water, then lay out a sheet of nori on your rolling mat. It has a smooth side and a rough side; lay it rough side up, with the long side parallel to you.
2.Lightly wet your hands and put a small handful of rice onto the nori. Gently spread the rice out to cover the sheet. Leave about 1 inch along the top edge free of rice.
3.Spoon about 2 tablespoons spicy chickpea filling along the bottom edge, side to side, along with a few cucumber sticks. All the veggies should only cover about one-third of the nori sheet.
4.Dry your hands, and pick up the bottom of the rolling mat. Roll it over the row of vegetables. Press tightly back toward you as you roll, and press down on the roll a bit. Do not squish, but make sure you are getting a tight roll.
5.Pick up the back end of the rolling mat. Dip a finger in the water, and run it along the top edge of the nori, where there is no rice. Then finish rolling, so the bare edge seals against the outside of the roll. Cover it back over with the mat, and gently compress the roll, just to help it seal.
6.Let your sushi roll sit for a few minutes for the nori to be softened by the rice, then cut into 6 to 8 slices and serve. Repeat to make 4 rolls.
7.Serve with a dipping bowl of tamari, some pickled ginger, and some wasabi.
Make ahead: Make double the rice if you want to make 4 of both this roll and the **Avocado Red Pepper Sushi Rolls** for a sushi party, or make one batch of rice and then 2 of each roll. Enjoy a piece of pickled ginger between as a palate cleanser.

Exquisite Banana, Apple, and Coconut Curry

Total time: 6 hours 10 minutes
Ingredients
1/2 cup of amaranth seeds
1 apple, cored and sliced
1 banana, sliced
1 1/2 cups of diced tomatoes
3 teaspoons of chopped parsley
1 green pepper, chopped
1 large white onion, peeled and diced
2 teaspoons of minced garlic
1 teaspoon of salt
1 teaspoon of ground cumin
2 1/2 tablespoons of curry powder
2 tablespoons of flour
2 bay leaves
1/2 cup of white wine
8 fluid ounce of coconut milk
1/2 cup of water

Directions:
Using a food processor place the apple, tomatoes, garlic and pulse it until it gets smooth but a little bit chunky.
Add this mixture to a 6-quarts slow cooker and add the remaining ingredients.
Stir until it mixes properly and cover the top.
Plug in the slow cooker; adjust the cooking time to 6 hours and let it cook on the low heat setting or until it is cooked thoroughly.
Add the seasoning and serve right away.

Hearty Vegetarian Lasagna Soup

Total time: 7 hours 20 minutes
Ingredients
12 ounces of lasagna noodles
4 cups of spinach leaves
2 cups of brown mushrooms, sliced
2 medium-sized zucchinis, stemmed and sliced
28 ounce of crushed tomatoes
1 medium-sized white onion, peeled and diced
2 teaspoon of minced garlic
1 tablespoon of dried basil
2 bay leaves
2 teaspoons of salt
1/8 teaspoon of red pepper flakes
2 teaspoons of ground black pepper
2 teaspoons of dried oregano
15-ounce of tomato sauce
6 cups of vegetable broth

Directions:
Grease a 6-quarts slow cooker and place all the ingredients in it except for the lasagna and spinach.
Cover the top, plug in the slow cooker; adjust the cooking time to 7 hours and let it cook on the low heat setting or until it is properly done.
In the meantime, cook the lasagna noodles in the boiling water for 7 to 10 minutes or until it gets soft.
Then drain and set it aside until the slow cooker is done cooking.
When it is done, add the lasagna noodles into the soup along with the spinach and continue cooking for 10 to 15 minutes or until the spinach leaves wilts.
Using a ladle, serving it in a bowl.

Inexpensive Bean and Spinach Enchiladas

Total time: 3 hours 5 minutes
Ingredients
2 cups of cooked black beans
1 cup of frozen corn
10 ounce of chopped spinach
Half of a medium-sized cucumber, peeled and sliced
6 cups of chopped lettuce
4 medium-sized radishes, peeled and cut into matchsticks
1/2 cup of cherry tomatoes, halved
1 teaspoon of salt, divided
1/2 teaspoon of ground black pepper, divided
1/2 teaspoon of ground cumin
3 1/2 cups of tomato salsa
2 cups of grated vegetarian cheddar cheese
8 corn tortillas, about 6-inch
3 tablespoons lime juice
2 tablespoons olive oil
Directions:
Place 1 cup of beans in a medium-sized bowl then ,using a fork mash them.
Then add the remaining beans, corn, spinach, 1/2 teaspoon of salt, 1/4 teaspoon of black pepper, 1 cup of cheddar cheese and stir until it mixes well.
Take a 6-quarts slow cooker and spread 2 cups of tomato salsa on the bottom.
Place the tortillas on a clean working space and proportionally top it with the prepared bean mixture, at least 1/2 cup.
Roll up the tortillas and place it into the slow cooker on top of the salsa, seam-side down.
Top it with the remaining tomato salsa, cheese and cover the top.
Plug in the slow cooker; adjust the cooking time to 3 hours and let it cook on the the low heat setting or until the cheese melts completely.
In the meantime, using a bowl, place the cucumber, lettuce, radish and tomatoes in it, sprinkle it with the lime juice, oil, the remaining of each salt and black pepper.
Toss to cover and serve this with the cooked enchiladas.

Delightful Coconut Vegetarian Curry

Total time: 4 hours 20 minutes
Ingredients
5 medium-sized potatoes, peeled and cut into 1-inch cubes
1/4 cup of curry powder
2 tablespoons of flour
1 tablespoon of chili powder
1/2 teaspoon of red pepper flakes
1/2 teaspoon of cayenne pepper
1 large green bell pepper, cut into strips
1 large red bell pepper, cut into strips
2 tablespoons of onion soup mix
14-ounce of coconut cream, unsweetened
3 cups of vegetable broth
2 medium-sized carrots, peeled and cut into matchstick
1 cup of green peas
1/4 cup of chopped cilantro
Directions:
Take a 6-quarts slow cooker, grease it with a non-stick cooking spray and place the potatoes pieces in the bottom.
Add the remaining ingredients except for the carrots, peas and cilantro.
Stir properly and cover the top.
Plug in the slow cooker; adjust the cooking time to 4 hours and let it cook on the low heat setting or until it cooks thoroughly.
When the cooking time is over, add the carrots to the curry and continue cooking for 30 minutes.
Then, add the peas and continue cooking for another 30 minutes or until the peas get tender.
Garnish it with cilantro and serve.

Creamy Sweet Potato & Coconut Curry

Total time: 6 hours 20 minutes

Ingredients

2 pounds of sweet potatoes, peeled and chopped
1/2 pound of red cabbage, shredded
2 red chilies, seeded and sliced
2 medium-sized red bell peppers, cored and sliced
2 large white onions, peeled and sliced
1 1/2 teaspoon of minced garlic
1 teaspoon of grated ginger
1/2 teaspoon of salt
1 teaspoon of paprika
1/2 teaspoon of cayenne pepper
2 tablespoons of peanut butter
4 tablespoons of olive oil
12-ounce of tomato puree
14 fluid ounce of coconut milk
1/2 cup of chopped coriander

Directions:

Place a large non-stick skillet pan over an average heat, add 1 tablespoon of oil and let it heat.

Then add the onion and cook for 10 minutes or until it gets soft.

Add the garlic, ginger, salt, paprika, cayenne pepper and continue cooking for 2 minutes or until it starts producing fragrance.

Transfer this mixture to a 6-quarts slow cooker, and reserve the pan.

In the pan, add 1 tablespoon of oil and let it heat.

Add the cabbage, red chili, bell pepper and cook it for 5 minutes.

Then transfer this mixture to the slow cooker and reserve the pan.

Add the remaining oil to the pan; the sweet potatoes in a single layer and cook it in 3 batches for 5 minutes or until it starts getting brown.

Add the sweet potatoes to the slow cooker, along with tomato puree, coconut milk and stir properly.

Cover the top, plug in the slow cooker; adjust the cooking time to 6 hours and let it cook on the low heat setting or until the sweet potatoes are tender.

When done, add the seasoning and pour it in the peanut butter.

Garnish it with coriander and serve.

Comforting Chickpea Tagine

Total time: 4 hours 15 minutes
Ingredients
14 ounce of cooked chickpeas
12 dried apricots
1 red bell pepper, cored and sliced
1 small butternut squash, peeled, cored and chopped
2 zucchini, stemmed and chopped
1 medium-sized white onion, peeled and chopped
1 teaspoon of minced garlic
1 teaspoon of ground ginger
1 1/2 teaspoon of salt
1 teaspoon of ground black pepper
1 teaspoon of ground cumin
2 teaspoon of paprika
1 teaspoon of harissa paste
2 teaspoon of honey
2 tablespoons of olive oil
1 pound of passata
1/4 cup of chopped coriander
Directions:
Take a 6-quarts slow cooker, grease it with a non-stick cooking spray and place the chickpeas, apricots, bell pepper, butternut squash, zucchini and onion into it.
Sprinkle it with salt, black pepper and set it aside until it is called for.
Place a large non-stick skillet pan over an average temperature of heat; add the oil, garlic, cumin and paprika.
Stir properly and cook for 1 minutes or until it starts producing fragrance.
Then pour in the harissa paste, honey, passata and boil the mixture.
When the mixture is done boiling, pour this mixture over the vegetables in the slow cooker and cover it with the lid.
Plug in the slow cooker; adjust the cooking time to 4 hours and let it cook on the high heat setting or until the vegetables gets tender.
When done, add the seasoning, garnish it with the coriander and serve right away.

Miso Ramen

Total time: 25 minutes
Ingredients
1/3 cup of spinach leaves (fresh)
1 cup of bean sprouts (fresh)
10 oz of ramen noodles (whole-wheat and dried)
½ cup of bamboo shoots (sliced, canned)
½ cup of corn kernels (fresh/ frozen)
8 cups of vegetable broth
2 tsp of instant dashi granules
1 tbsp of tamari sauce to taste
4 tbsp of miso paste
1 green onion (chopped finely)
Directions:
Boil, drain and cut spinach, 1 minute.
Boil, drain and remove the sprouts from the beans.
Over medium heat, boil the ramen noodles and cook as directed on the package.
In 4 wide servings bowl, divide the noodles, bamboo shoots, corn kernels, bean sprouts and spinach.
Pour the stock, instant dashi granules, and tamari sauce in a medium pot. Boil, cool and stir in the miso paste.
Pour the mixture into the ramen bowl, garnish with the green onion and serve immediately.

Noodles with Sticky Tofu

Total time: 25 minutes
Ingredients
½ large size cucumber
2 tbsp of pure date sugar
100ml of wine vinegar (rice)
100ml of olive oil
200g pack of tofu (fir, cut into cubes)
2 tbsp of maple syrup
4 tbsp of white miso paste
30g of sesame seeds (white)
250g soba noodles (dried)
2 spring onions, (shredded, garnish)
Directions:
Cut thin ribbons off the cucumber using a peeler, leaving behind the seeds. In a tub, place the ribbons and reserve. Heat the date sugar, ¼ tsp salt, 100 ml of water and vinegar gently in a casserole over medium heat for 3 to 5 minutes until the date sugar is dissolved, then pour over the cucumbers and leave to pickle in the fridge while preparing the tofu.
In a large, non-stick frying pan, warm all but 1 tbsp of the oil over medium heat until bubbles start to come to the surface. Add the tofu and fry for 7-10 minutes until the tofu is uniformly golden brown, turning halfway. Remove the tofu from the pan and place on paper to drain grease.
Whisk together the pure maple syrup and miso in a small bowl. Place the sesame seeds on a plate.
Brush the tofu with the sticky pure maple syrup sauce and sprinkle with the sesame seeds.
Warm the noodles as instructed by the box, then drain and rinse under cold water.
Return the frying pan to heat with a little oil, throw in the noodles, and toss.
In 4 medium bowls, divide the noodles, tofu, pickled cucumber, spring onion, and some of the miso sauce.
Serve immediately.

Almond Butter Tofu Stir- fry

Total time: 65 minutes
Ingredients
Tofu
2 x 12 oz package of tofu (extra firm and pressed)
Marinade
8 tbsp of tamari sauce
4 tbsp of sesame oil (divided)
4 tbsp of almond butter
4 tbsp of lime (squeezed)
4 tsp of chili garlic sauce
6 tbsp of maple syrup
Directions:
Set the oven to 400 degrees F and use baking paper to line a baking tray.
Arrange the tofu on the baking sheet and cook in the oven until golden brown, and cooked through, 10 to 15 minutes.
In a medium bowl, mix half of the tamari, sesame oil, almond butter, lime juice, garlic chili sauce and maple syrup to a medium bowl.
Add the tofu, toss well, and sit for 5 minutes.
Heat a little oil in a medium skillet and fry the tofu on both sides until golden brown, 1 to 2 minutes.
Serve the tofu with steamed spinach.

Vegetable Farro Harvest Bowl

Total time: 65 minutes

Ingredients

16 oz of Brussels sprouts (halved)
1 sweet potato (diced)
1 red pepper (cut into cubes)
2 tbsp of olive oil
1/2 tsp of cinnamon (ground)
1 red onion (halved and quartered)
3 ½ cups of water
1 cup of farro
½ cup of basil (fresh)
2 tbsp of olive oil
1 tsp of salt
2 tbsp of wine vinegar (red)
1 clove of garlic
Salt and black pepper to taste
2 tsp of mustard (Dijon)

Directions:

Set the oven to 400 F.

Heat the olive oil in a medium skillet and cook the Brussels sprouts, sweet potatoes, red pepper, salt, cinnamon and red onion until softened, 30 minutes.

Meanwhile, place the water and farro in a pan. Boil, cover the lid, and simmer for 30 minutes or until the farro softens and the water is absorbed. Fluff and set aside.

In a medium bowl, mix the basil, olive oil, wine vinegar, garlic cover, salt, pepper and Dijon mustard until smooth. Divide the vegetables, farro, and dressing into 4 medium bowls, and serve.

Vegan Garlic Slaw Burger

Total time: 45 minutes
Ingredients
Veggie Burger/ Patties
½ cup of green lentils (uncooked)
2 cloves of garlic
¼ cup of onion (white)
1 medium size carrot (chopped roughly)
½ tsp of sea salt
½ tsp of chili flakes (crushed)
1 tsp of tamari sauce
1 tsp of sriracha or hot sauce
1/3 cup of panko breadcrumbs
2 tbsp flax egg
1 tsp sesame oil
4 whole-wheat burger buns, halved
Slaw
1 tbsp of plant-based yogurt
1 tbsp of tofu mayonnaise
1 tsp of sesame oil
1 tsp of tamari sauce
1 tsp of sambal chili sauce
3 tbsp of rice vinegar
3 minis of cucumbers (julienned finely)
2 medium size carrots (julienned finely)
2 green onions (sliced thinly)
2 tbsp of sesame seeds (toasted)

Directions:
Veggie burger/ patties
Add all the burgers ingredients except for the oil and bread into a food processor and blend until smooth. Form 4 to 6 patties from the mixture.
Heat 2 tbsp of sesame oil in a medium skillet and fry the patties on both sides until golden brown and compacted, 10 minutes.
Slaw
In a medium bowl, mix the slaw's ingredients and set aside to combine flavors for 10 minutes.
To serve, place the burger patties between the burger buns, top with the slaw and serve immediately.

Easy Vegan Samosa Pot- Pie

Total time: 45 minutes
Ingredients
1 tbsp of vegetable oil
1 large size onion (diced)
3 cloves of garlic (minced)
2 medium size potatoes (diced and peeled)
150g of frozen green peas (defrosted)
2 tbsp of curry powder
1 tsp of chili powder
1 tbsp of cilantro (dried)
400g soy (frozen, mince)
Salt and pepper to taste
1 pack of whole-wheat filo pastry (defrosted)
2 tbsp of vegetable oil
 Directions:
Set the oven to 350 F.
Heat the olive oil in a medium pot and sauté the onion, garlic, potatoes, and cook until softened, 10 minutes.
Mix in the green peas, curry powder, chili powder, cilantro, soy, salt, and pepper. Cook for 2 to 3 minutes or until the green peas warm through.
Spoon the mixture into 4 medium ramekins.
Roll out the filo pastry, divide into 4 pieces and spread over the ramekins.
Brush with a little oil, place on a baking sheet, and bake in the oven for 20 to 25 minutes or until the pastry is golden brown.
Remove the ramekins from the oven, allow cooling, and serve warm.

Seitan Spiced Meatballs

Total time: 75 minutes
Ingredients
1 tbsp flax egg
2 tbsp of olive oil
6 large size of garlic cloves (minced finely)
1 small size of onion (minced finely)
1 tsp of sea salt
1 tbsp of chili powder
1 tsp of cumin (ground)
1 tsp of fennel seed (ground)
1 tsp of black pepper
1 ¼ cup of textured vegetable protein (dry, TVP)
½ tbsp of Italian seasoning
¼ tsp of red pepper (crushed)
1 cup of water
2 tbsp of tamari sauce
2 tbsp of vegan parmesan cheese
½ cup of wheat gluten (vital or seitan)
2 tbsp coconut oil
Directions:
Combine all the ingredients in a medium bowl until well combined and form 2-inch size balls from the mixture.
Heat the oil in a medium skillet and fry the meatballs on until golden brown on all sides. Meanwhile, making sure they are cooked within.
Transfer to serving bowls and serve warm.

Potato Tofu Scramble

Total time: 15 minutes
Ingredients
6 small size of fingerling potatoes
16 pcs of mushrooms
2 small size of shallot
4 tbsp of oil (divided)
10oz tofu (dry)
½ tsp of turmeric
2 tbsp of nutritional yeast
4 cups of spinach
½ tsp of salt
Pinch black pepper
Directions:
Split the potatoes into ¼- inch cubes. Cut the mushroom into quarters, and chop the shallot in half moon shape.
In a frying pan, heat a tbsp of oil over medium heat. Cook in the potatoes until softened and turned brown, 7 minutes.
Mix in the mushrooms, shallots and cook for at least 3 minutes or until the mushrooms shallots soften. Use the spoon to move the mixture to the side of the pan.
Add 1 tbsp of oil if desire or needed and crumble in the tofu into the saucepan. Cook until golden brown and season with the turmeric and nutritional yeast, 4 minutes.
Mix all the ingredients and work in the spinach. Cook until wilted, 3 minutes.

Nutty Stuffed Squash

Total time: 60 minutes
Ingredients
3 tbsp of butter (vegan)
3 cloves of garlic (minced)
¾ tsp of sea salt
2 medium size yellow onions (chopped finely)
1 tbsp of fresh sage (chopped)
2 tbsp flax egg
1/3 cup of plant-based yogurt
½ cup of parmesan cheese (freshly shredded)
2 squash (halved lengthwise, seeded)
Mixed toasted nuts for topping
Directions:
Set the oven to 350 F.
Melt the butter over medium - high heat in a saucepan. Cook in the garlic, onion, and season with salt until softened, 3 minutes. Set aside.
In a medium bowl, mix the flax egg, yogurt, onion mixture, and parmesan in a mixing container. Split the filling between the squash halves, spread with more parmesan, and bake until soft and brown, 45 minutes.
Remove from the oven, top with some nuts and serve warm.

Smoked Tofu and Watercress Cannelloni

Total time: 45 minutes
Ingredients
Vegetable oil or olive oil
2 red onions (diced and peeled)
2 cloves of garlic (chopped finely)
2 tsp of thyme (dried)
Salt and pepper to taste
225g of spinach
225g of watercress
2 packs of tofu (smoked)
1 tsp of paprika (smoked)
20 tubes of cannelloni pasta (whole-wheat and dried)
1 cup of tomatoes sauce
Directions:
Set the oven at 350 F and grease a baking sheet with cooking spray.
In a large pot, heat the oil and sauté the onion, garlic, thyme, and season with salt and black pepper, 3 minutes.
Mix in the spinach and watercress and allow wilting, 3 minutes.
Add the tofu, paprika, and cook until the tofu warms through, 3 minutes.
Spoon the mixture into a piping bag, tear open a wide hole and press the mixture into the cannelloni.
Arrange the pasta in the baking dish and pour the tomato sauce on top. Season with salt, black pepper, and scatter some cashew cheese on top,
Bake in the oven until the cheese melts and the pasta cooks, 35 minutes.

Grilled Cauliflower Steak with Hummus and Quinoa

Total time: 25 minutes
Ingredients
150g of cauliflower
60g of quinoa
40g of edamame beans
25g of hummus
20g of hemp seeds
Coriander leaves (for garnish)
¼ lemon (for garnish)
Directions:
Boil the whole cauliflower for 10 to 12 minutes.
Allow cooling and cut the cauliflower into steak style pieces.
Preheat a grill to medium heat and brown the cauliflower steaks on both sides, 5 minutes.
Bring water to the boil in a casserole, add quinoa and cook for 10 minutes. After, fluff and set aside.
In a cup, mix the olive oil, salt, and edamame beans.
Layer the hummus over a sheet and cover with the mixture of quinoa. Put the grilled cauliflower on top, sprinkle with the seeds of hemp and dust the leaves of coriander and voila!

Chirashi Grain Bowl

Total time: 25 minutes
Ingredients
1 tbsp of olive oil (extra virgin)
1 small size of carrot (julienned, sliced thinly)
 1 small size ginger (julienned, peeled)
1 tsp of sesame seeds
½ tsp of toasted sesame oil
2 tbsp of vegetable oil
1 cup shiitake mushrooms (finely chopped)
2 tsp of tamari sauce
½ tsp of pure date sugar (granulated)
1 tsp of sake
1 plum tomato (sliced in bite size)
1 tbsp of white miso paste
1 tbsp of olive oil (extra virgin)
½ cup of baby spinach (chopped finely)
1 cup of brown rice or quinoa
3 tbsp of rice vinegar
2 stalks of scallions (chopped finely)
shredded nori (optional)
Directions:
In a medium saucepan, heat the olive oil over medium heat and sauté the carrots and ginger until softened, 5 minutes.
Season with some salt and mix in the sesame seeds and sesame oil. Transfer to a plate and set aside.
Heat the vegetable oil in the skillet and cook in the shiitake mushrooms until softened. Add the tamari sauce, date sugar, sake and cook until all of the liquid has absorbed. Place on a plate and reserve.
Place the tomatoes with miso paste and extra virgin olive oil in a small bowl. Blend well.
Heat the rice or quinoa and pour over the rice vinegar until completely covered.
Divide all the cooked foods and remaining ingredients between 4 serving bowls and serve.

Chickpea Sweetcorn Veggie Burger

Total time: 40 minutes
Ingredients
Olive oil (extra virgin)
1 onion (chopped finely)
1 clove of garlic (chopped finely)
1 tsp of coriander (ground)
200g of sweetcorn (cooked)
400g of chickpeas (tinned, drained, rinsed)
1 tbsp of parsley (chopped)
100g of whole-wheat breadcrumbs
60g of flour (spelt)
1 tbsp flax egg
To coat the burgers
40g of flour (spelt)
1 tsp of cumin (ground)
Directions:
Preheat the oven to 350 F.
Heat the olive oil in a medium saucepan and sauté the onion until softened, 3 minutes. Add the garlic, coriander and cook for 1 to 2 minutes. Set aside.
In a medium bowl, mash and mix the chickpeas, parsley, onion mixture, breadcrumbs, flour, and flax egg.
Blend sweetcorn, chickpeas and parsley and pulse until well mixed.
Bring the mixture of onions, breadcrumbs, flour, flax egg and mix. From 4 to 6 patties from the mixture and place on a baking sheet. Bake in the oven until golden brown and compacted, 10 to 15 minutes.
Remove the sheet from the oven and set aside to cool slightly.
In a shallow plate, mix the flour and cumin powder, and coat the burgers in the mixture.
Heat a little olive oil in a medium skillet and fry the patties on both sides until crusty, 3 to 4 minutes.
Place the patties between the burger buns.
Best served with hummus, garden greens, and tofu mayonnaise.
Serve warm.

Grilled Breaded Tofu Steaks

Total time: 25 minutes
Ingredients
350g of tofu (extra-firm)
4 cloves of garlic
1 tbsp of dijon mustard
1 tbsp of maple syrup
2 tbsp of tomato paste
1 tbsp of tamari sauce
¼ tsp of black pepper
1 tbsp of water
½ cup of panko breadcrumbs (whole wheat)
2 tbsp of olive oil
A BBQ sauce for dipping (your choice)
Directions:
Press the tofu between two pieces of parchment paper and cut into steaks.
In the medium bowl, mix the garlic powder, Dijon mustard, maple syrup, tomato paste, tamari sauce, and black pepper. Add the tofu, mix well and allow marinating for 10 minutes.
Pour the breadcrumbs into a shallow plate and coat the tofu slightly in the crumbs.
Heat the olive oil in a medium skillet and fry on both sides until golden brown and cooked within.
Serve the tofu with the BBQ sauce.

Nourishing Curried Lentil and Sweet Potato Bowl

Total time: 30 minutes
Ingredients
Lentils
1 cup yellow lentils
Potatoes
2 tbsp of avocado oil
1 large size of sweet potato (cut into rounds, skin- on)
¼ tsp of sea salt
Cauliflower Rice
1 tbsp of water
1 tbsp of olive oil
A pinch of sea salt
½ tsp curry powder
1 head of cauliflower (grated)
Kale
1 bundle of organic kale (chopped)
Directions:
Cook the lentils in 1 cup of water in a medium pot over medium heat until softened, 10 minutes.
Set the oven to 375 F and line a baking tray with parchment paper.
In a medium bowl, mix the avocado oil, sweet potatoes, salt, and spread on the baking sheet. Bake in the oven until the sweet potatoes soften, 15 to 20 minutes.
Meanwhile, combine the cauliflower ingredients in a safe microwave bowl and steam in the microwave until softened, 1 minute.
Also, heat 1 tsp of avocado oil in a medium skillet and sauté the kale until wilted.
In a medium bowl, divide the lentils, sweet potatoes, cauliflower rice, kale, and serve warm.

Curried Potato and Lentil Soup Pot

Total time: 40 minutes
Ingredients
2 tbsp of olive oil
½ cup of carrots (diced)
1 cup onion (yellow, diced)
½ cup of celery (diced)
1 tbsp of garlic (minced)
1 tsp of pure date sugar
1 tbsp of wine vinegar (red)
1 tsp of sea salt
3 tbsp of curry powder
1 tsp of ginger (fresh, grated)
1 lb. of green lentils
8 cups of vegetable broth (divided)
14.5 oz tomatoes petite (diced)
1 lb. red potatoes (cut into an inch/pcs)
Directions:
Heat the olive oil in a medium pot and sauté the carrots, onions and celery until softened, 5 minutes.
Mix in the garlic, date sugar, vinegar, salt, curry powder and ginger. Cook for 1 minute, mix well to blend.
After, add the lentils, 6 cups of broth, tomatoes and potatoes. Mix well.
Cover the lid and cook for 6 to 7 minutes or until the potatoes soften.
Adjust the taste with salt, black pepper, and dish the soup.
Serve immediately.

Vegan Teriyaki Tofu

Total time: 25 minutes
Ingredients
3 tsp of olive oil
4 tbsp of tamari sauce
2 tbsp of pure date sugar
A pinch of ginger (ground)
2 tbsp of mirin
½ tbsp of oil (rapeseed)
2 medium zucchinis (sliced horizontally/ strips)
200g of broccoli (tender stem)
350g of tofu (block, very firm, cut into slices)
Black sesame seeds for garnish
Directions:
In a medium bowl, mix 1 tsp olive oil, tamari sauce, pure date sugar, mirin and ginger, and rub it all over tofu slices. Place them in a big dish and pour over any remaining marinade. Leave to settle for an hour.
After preheat a grill pan over medium-high heat.
In a medium bowl, mix the remaining olive oil and rapeseed oil. Brush both sides of the zucchini and broccoli with the oil and cook on both sides until tender, 5 to 7 minutes.
Grill the tofu slices on both sides until brown and crispy on the edges, 5 minutes.
Serve the tofu with the vegetables.

Sesame Eggplant & Almond Butter Tofu Bowl

Total time: 20 minutes
Ingredients
Tofu
8 oz of tofu (extra firm)
2 tbsp of sesame oil
3 tbsp of cornstarch
Sauce
1 tbsp of sesame oil
1 tbsp of tamari sauce
1 tbsp of lime (squeezed)
2 tbsp of almond butter (salted)
1 medium size of Birdseye chili (crushed)
2 tbsp of maple syrup
Eggplant
1 tbsp of sesame oil (toasted)
2 medium size of Japanese eggplants (skin- on, stem removed, cut in 1-inch pieces)
1 tbsp of maple syrup
1 tbsp of tamari sauce
Directions:
Wrap the tofu in a clean towel. Place a heavy lid on top for 10 minutes to press out the excess liquid. Cut into cubes and set aside.
For the sauce: in a medium bowl, whisk the sesame oil, tamari, lime juice, almond butter, crushed chili and maple syrup to prepare the tofu sauce in a medium bowl and set aside.
For the tofu: heat 2 tbsp of sesame oil in a medium skillet, coat the tofu with some cornstarch and fry in the oil on both sides until golden brown.
Mix in the almond butter sauce and cook for 2 to 3 minutes. Transfer to a plate and set aside.
For the eggplant: heat 1 tbsp of sesame oil in a medium skillet over medium heat and cook in the eggplant until softened.
Top with the maple syrup, tamari sauce, and cook until light brown and softened, 2 to 3 minutes.
Serve the eggplant and tofu with cooked white rice.

Summer Pistou

Total time: 25 minutes
Ingredients
1 tbsp of oil (rapeseed)
2 leeks (sliced finely)
1 large size of zucchini (diced finely)
2 cups of vegetable stock (boiling)
3 tomatoes (chopped)
200g of beans (green, chopped)
400g of haricot beans (drained)
3 cloves of garlic (chopped finely)
40g of vegan Parmesan cheese
small pack of basil
Directions:
In a medium saucepan, heat olive oil for 5 minutes and sauté the leeks and zucchini. Pour in the stock, add half tomatoes, green beans, three-quarters of haricot beans, and cook for 5 to 8 minutes until vegetables are soft.
In a food processor, blend the remaining tomatoes, beans; garlic and basil until fluffy, and then add the vegan Parmesan.
Pour the sauce into the soup, simmer for 2 minutes, and serve afterwards.

Lentil Lasagna

Total time: 75 minutes
Ingredients
1 tbsp of olive oil
1 onion (chopped)
1 celery (chopped, stick)
1 carrot (chopped)
1 clove of garlic (crushed)
1 tbsp of corn flour
2 cans of 400g lentils (drained, rinsed)
400g of tomato (chopped)
1 tsp of ketchup (mushroom)
1 tsp of vegetable stock (powder)
1 tsp of oregano (chopped)
2 cauliflower (heads, cut into florets and steamed)
2 tbsp of soya milk (unsweetened)
A pinch of grated nutmeg (freshly)
9 egg-free lasagna sheets (dried)

Directions:
In a medium saucepan, heat the olive oil and sauté the onion, celery and carrot until softened, 5 minutes. Add the garlic, cook for 2 more minutes, and stir in the corn flour and lentils.
Pour tomatoes, mushroom ketchup, stock powder, oregano and some seasoning. Bring to a boil for 15 minutes.
In a blender, process the cauliflower, soya milk, and nutmeg until smooth.
Preheat the oven to 350 F.
Lay over the base, a ceramic casserole dish, a third of the lentil mixture then, fill with a single layer of lasagna sheet. Top with another third of the lentil mixture, then spread over a third of the cauliflower purée, followed by a pasta layer. Finish with the last third of lentils and lasagna, then the remainder of the purée.
Cover with foil and bake for 35 to 45 minutes.
Remove the dish, foil, and allow cooling for 2 minutes.
Serve warm.

Super tasty Vegetarian Chili

Total time: 2 hours 10 minutes
Ingredients
16-ounce of vegetarian baked beans
16 ounce of cooked chickpeas
16 ounce of cooked kidney beans
15 ounce of cooked corn
1 medium-sized green bell pepper, cored and chopped
2 stalks of celery, peeled and chopped
12 ounce of chopped tomatoes
1 medium-sized white onion, peeled and chopped
1 teaspoon of minced garlic
1 teaspoon of salt
1 tablespoon of red chili powder
1 tablespoon of dried oregano
1 tablespoon of dried basil
1 tablespoon of dried parsley
18-ounce of black bean soup
4-ounce of tomato puree

Directions:
Take a 6-quarts slow cooker, grease it with a non-stick cooking spray and place all the ingredients into it.
Stir properly and cover the top.
Plug in the slow cooker; adjust the cooking time to 2 hours and let it cook on the high heat setting or until it is cooked thoroughly.
Serve right away.

Vegetable Soup

Total time: 6 hours 30 minutes

Ingredients

1/4 cup of vegetable shortening
2 cups of all-purpose flour, leveled
1/2 cup of barley, uncooked
16 ounce of diced tomatoes
2 medium-sized potatoes, peeled and cubed
16 ounce of frozen mixed vegetables
1 large white onion, peeled and diced
1 1/2 teaspoon of minced garlic
6 cups of vegetable broth
1/2 teaspoon of salt
1/2 teaspoon of dried basil
1/2 teaspoon of ground black pepper
1 teaspoon of dried oregano
1 teaspoon of dried parsley
1 bay leaf
6 1/4 cup of vegetable broth

Directions:

Take a 6 quarts slow cooker, grease it with a non-stick cooking spray and add all the ingredients except for flour, vegetable shortening and reserve 1/4 cup of vegetable broth.

Stir properly and cover the top.

Plug in the slow cooker; adjust the cooking time to 6 hours and let it cook on the low heat setting or until it is cooked thoroughly.

In the meantime, place the flour, shortening in a food processor and pulse it until the mixture resembles crumbs. Then gradually mix the reserved 1/4 cup of vegetable broth until the smooth dough comes together.

Transfer the dough to a clean space filled with flour and roll it into the 1/8 thick dough.

Using a sharp knife cut the dough into small squares and put them in the slow cooker when 6 hours of cooking time is over.

Continue cooking for 1 hour at the high heat setting or until the dumplings are soft.

Scoop it into the serving bowls and serve.

Tastiest Barbecued Tofu and Vegetables

Total time: 4 hours 15 minutes
Ingredients
14-ounce of extra-firm tofu, pressed and drained
2 medium-sized zucchini, stemmed and diced
1/2 large green bell pepper, cored and cubed
3 stalks of broccoli stalks
8 ounce of sliced water chestnuts
1 small white onion, peeled and minced
1 1/2 teaspoon of minced garlic
2 teaspoons of minced ginger
1 1/2 teaspoon of salt
1/8 teaspoon of ground black pepper
1/4 teaspoon of crushed red pepper
1/4 teaspoon of five spice powder
2 teaspoons of molasses
1 tablespoon of whole-grain mustard
1/4 teaspoon of vegan Worcestershire sauce
8 ounces of tomato sauce
1/4 cup of hoisin sauce
1 tablespoon of soy sauce
2 tablespoons of apple cider vinegar
2 tablespoons of water
Directions:
Take a 6-quarts slow cooker, grease it with a non-stick cooking spray and set it aside until it is required.
Place a medium-sized non-stick skillet pan over an average heat, add the oil and let it heat.
Cut the tofu into 1/2 inch pieces and add it to the skillet pan in a single layer.
Cook for 3 minutes per sides and then transfer it to the prepared slow cooker.
When the tofu turns brown, place it into the pan, add the onion, garlic, ginger and cook for 3 to 5 minutes or until the onions are softened.
Add the remaining ingredients into the pan except for the vegetables which are the broccoli stalks, zucchini, bell pepper and water chestnuts.
Stir until it mixes properly and cook for 2 minutes or until the mixture starts bubbling.
Transfer this mixture into the slow cooker and stir properly.
Cover the top, plug in the slow cooker; adjust the cooking time to 3 hours and let it cook on the high heat setting or until it is cooked thoroughly.
In the meantime, trim the broccoli stalks and cut it into 1/4 inch pieces.
When the tofu is cooked thoroughly, put it into the slow cooker; add the broccoli stalks and the remaining vegetables.
Stir until it mixes properly and then return the top to cover it.
Continue cooking for 1 hour at the high heat setting or until the vegetables are tender.
Serve right away with rice.

Savory Spanish Rice

Total time: 3 hours 10 minutes
Ingredients
1 cup of long grain rice, uncooked
1/2 cup of chopped green bell pepper
14 ounce of diced tomatoes
1/2 cup of chopped white onion
1 teaspoon of minced garlic
1/2 teaspoon of salt
1 teaspoon of red chili powder
1 teaspoon of ground cumin
4-ounce of tomato puree
8 fluid ounce of water
Directions:
Grease a 6-quarts slow cooker with a non-stick cooking spray and add all the ingredients into it.
Stir properly and cover the top.
Plug in the slow cooker; adjust the cooking time to 5 hours and let it cook on the high heat setting or until the rice absorbs all the liquid.
Serve right away.

Chapter 8: Snacks Recipes

Beetroot Hummus

Total time: 70 minutes
 Ingredients
15 ounces cooked chickpeas
3 small beets
1 teaspoon minced garlic
1/2 teaspoon smoked paprika
1 teaspoon of sea salt
1/4 teaspoon red chili flakes
2 tablespoons olive oil
1 lemon, juiced
2 tablespoon tahini
1 tablespoon chopped almonds
1 tablespoon chopped cilantro
Directions:
Drizzle oil over beets, season with salt, then wrap beets in a foil and bake for 60 minutes at 425 degrees F until tender.
When done, let beet cool for 10 minutes, then peel and dice them and place them in a food processor.
Add remaining ingredients and pulse for 2 minutes until smooth, tip the hummus in a bowl, drizzle with some more oil, and then serve straight away.

Carrot and Sweet Potato Fritters

Total time: 18 minutes
Ingredients
1/3 cup quinoa flour
1½ cups shredded sweet potato
1 cup grated carrot
1/3 teaspoon ground black pepper
2/3 teaspoon salt
2 teaspoons curry powder
2 flax eggs
2 tablespoons coconut oil
Directions:
Place all the ingredients in a bowl, except for oil, stir well until combined and then shape the mixture into ten small patties
Take a large pan, place it over medium-high heat, add oil and when it melts, add patties in it and cook for 3 minutes per side until browned.
Serve straight away

Black Bean Lime Dip

Total time: 11 minutes
Ingredients
15.5 ounces cooked black beans
1 teaspoon minced garlic
½ of a lime, juiced
1 inch of ginger, grated
1/3 teaspoon salt
1/3 teaspoon ground black pepper
1 tablespoon olive oil
Directions:
Take a frying pan, add oil and when hot, add garlic and ginger and cook for 1 minute until fragrant.
Then add beans, splash with some water and fry for 3 minutes until hot.
Season beans with salt and black pepper, drizzle with lime juice, then remove the pan from heat and mash the beans until smooth pasta comes together.
Serve the dip with whole-grain breadsticks or vegetables.

Apple and Honey Toast

Total time: 5 minutes
 Ingredients
½ of a small apple, cored, sliced
1 slice of whole-grain bread, toasted
1 tablespoon honey
2 tablespoons hummus
1/8 teaspoon cinnamon
Directions:
Spread hummus on one side of the toast, top with apple slices and then drizzle with honey.
Sprinkle cinnamon on it and then serve straight away.

Thai Snack Mix

Total time: 115 minutes
 Ingredients
5 cups mixed nuts
1 teaspoon onion powder
1 cup chopped dried pineapple
1 cup pumpkin seed
2 teaspoons paprika
1/2 teaspoon ground black pepper
1 teaspoon of sea salt
1/4 cup coconut sugar
1/2 teaspoon red chili powder
1 tablespoon red pepper flakes
1 teaspoon garlic powder
1/2 tablespoon red curry powder
2 tablespoons soy sauce
2 tablespoons coconut oil
Directions:
Switch on the slow cooker, add all the ingredients in it except for dried pineapple and red pepper flakes, stir until combined and cook for 90 minutes at high heat setting, stirring every 30 minutes.
When done, spread the nut mixture on a baking sheet lined with parchment paper and let it cool.
Then spread dried pineapple on top, sprinkle with red pepper flakes and serve.

Zucchini Fritters

Total time: 16 minutes
Ingredients
1/2 cup quinoa flour
3 1/2 cups shredded zucchini
1/2 cup chopped scallions
1/3 teaspoon ground black pepper
1 teaspoon salt
2 tablespoons coconut oil
2 flax eggs
Directions:
Squeeze moisture from the zucchini by wrapping it in a cheesecloth and then transfer it to a bowl.
Add remaining ingredients, except for oil, stir until combined and then shape the mixture into twelve patties.
Take a skillet pan, place it over medium-high heat, add oil and when hot, add patties and cook for 3 minutes per side until brown.
Serve the patties with favorite vegan sauce.

Quinoa Broccoli Tots

Total time: 30 minutes
Ingredients
2 tablespoons quinoa flour
2 cups steamed and chopped broccoli florets
1/2 cup nutritional yeast
1 teaspoon garlic powder
1 teaspoon miso paste
2 flax eggs
2 tablespoons hummus
Directions:
Place all the ingredients in a bowl, stir until well combined, and then shape the mixture into sixteen small balls.
Arrange the balls on a baking sheet lined with parchment paper, spray with oil and bake at 400 degrees F for 20 minutes until brown, turning halfway.
When done, let the tots cool for 10 minutes and then serve straight away.

Spicy Roasted Chickpeas

Total time: 30 minutes
Ingredients
30 ounces cooked chickpeas
½ teaspoon salt
2 teaspoons mustard powder
½ teaspoon cayenne pepper
2 tablespoons olive oil
Directions:
Place all the ingredients in a bowl and stir until well coated and then spread the chickpeas in an even layer on a baking sheet greased with oil.
Bake the chickpeas for 20 minutes at 400 degrees F until golden brown and crispy and then serve straight away.

Nacho Kale Chips

Total time: 14 hours 10 minutes
Ingredients
2 bunches of curly kale
2 cups cashews, soaked, drained
1/2 cup chopped red bell pepper
1 teaspoon garlic powder
1 teaspoon salt
2 tablespoons red chili powder
1/2 teaspoon smoked paprika
1/2 cup nutritional yeast
1 teaspoon cayenne
3 tablespoons lemon juice
3/4 cup water
Directions:
Place all the ingredients except for kale in a food processor and pulse for 2 minutes until smooth.
Place kale in a large bowl, pour in the blended mixture, mix until coated, and dehydrate for 14 hours at 120 degrees F until crispy.
If dehydrator is not available, spread kale between two baking sheets and bake for 90 minutes at 225 degrees F until crispy, flipping halfway.
When done, let chips cool for 15 minutes and then serve.

Marinated Mushrooms

Total time: 17 minutes
Ingredients
1/4 teaspoon dried thyme
1/2 teaspoon sea salt
1/2 teaspoon dried basil
1/2 teaspoon red pepper flakes
1/4 teaspoon dried oregano
1/2 teaspoon maple syrup
1 teaspoon minced garlic
1/4 cup apple cider vinegar
1/4 cup and 1 teaspoon olive oil
2 tablespoons chopped parsley
12 ounces small button mushrooms
Directions:
Take a skillet pan, place it over medium-high heat, add 1 teaspoon oil and when hot, add mushrooms and cook for 5 minutes until golden brown.
Meanwhile, prepare the marinade and for this, place remaining ingredients in a bowl and whisk until combined. When mushrooms have cooked, transfer them into the bowl of marinade and toss until well coated.
Serve straight away

Hummus Quesadillas

Total time: 20 minutes
Ingredients
1 tortilla, whole wheat
1/4 cup diced roasted red peppers
1 cup baby spinach
1/3 teaspoon minced garlic
¼ teaspoon salt
¼ teaspoon ground black pepper
1/4 teaspoon olive oil
1/4 cup hummus
Oil as needed
Directions:
Place a large pan over medium heat, add oil and when hot, add red peppers and garlic, season with salt and black pepper and cook for 3 minutes until sauté.
Then stir in spinach, cook for 1 minute, remove the pan from heat and transfer the mixture in a bowl.
Prepare quesadilla and for this, spread hummus on one-half of the tortilla, then spread spinach mixture on it, cover the filling with the other half of the tortilla and cook in a pan for 3 minutes per side until browned.
When done, cut the quesadilla into wedges and serve.

Nacho Cheese Sauce

Total time: 15 minutes

 Ingredients

3 tablespoons flour
1/4 teaspoon garlic salt
1/4 teaspoon salt
1/2 teaspoon cumin
1/4 teaspoon paprika
1 teaspoon red chili powder
1/8 teaspoon cayenne powder
1 cup vegan cashew yogurt
1 1/4 cups vegetable broth

Directions

Take a small saucepan, place it over medium heat, pour in vegetable broth, and bring it to a boil.

Then whisk together flour and yogurt, add to the boiling broth, stir in all the spices, switch heat to medium-low level and cook for 5 minutes until thickened.

Serve straight away.

Salted Almonds

Total time: 25 minutes

Ingredients

2 cups almonds
4 tablespoons salt
1 cup boiling water

Directions:

Stir the salt into the boiling water in a pan, then add almonds in it and let them soak for 20 minutes.

Then drain the almonds, spread them in an even layer on a baking sheet lined with baking paper and sprinkle with salt.

Roast the almonds for 20 minutes at 300 degrees F, then cool them for 10 minutes and serve.

Pumpkin Cake Pops

Total time: 20 minutes

 Ingredients

1 cup coconut flour
¼ teaspoon cinnamon
1/4 cup coconut sugar
1/4 cup chocolate chips, unsweetened
3/4 cup pumpkin puree

Directions:

Place all the ingredients in a bowl, except for chocolate chips, stir until incorporated, and then fold in chocolate chips until combined.

Shape the mixture into small balls, then place them on a cookie sheet greased with oil and bake for 10 minutes at 350 degrees F until done.

Let the balls cool completely and then serve.

Watermelon Pizza

Total time: 10 minutes
 Ingredients
1/2 cup strawberries, halved
1/2 cup blueberries
1 watermelon
1/2 cup raspberries
1 cup of coconut yogurt
1/2 cup pomegranate seeds
1/2 cup cherries
Maple syrup as needed
Directions:
Cut watermelon into 3-inch thick slices, then spread yogurt on one side, leaving some space in the edges and then top evenly with fruits and drizzle with maple syrup.
Cut the watermelon into wedges and then serve.

Rosemary Popcorn

Total time: 20 minutes
Ingredients
1/2 cup popcorn kernels
1/2 teaspoon sea salt
1 tablespoon and 1/2 teaspoon minced rosemary
3 tablespoons unsalted vegan butter
1/4 cup olive oil
1/3 teaspoon ground black pepper
Directions:
Take a pot, place it over medium-low heat, add oil and when it melts, add four kernels and wait until they sizzle.
Then add remaining kernel, toss until coated, add 1 tablespoon minced rosemary, shut the pot with the lid, and shake the kernels until popped completely.
Once all the kernels have popped, transfer them in a bowl, cook remaining rosemary into melted butter, then drizzle this mixture over popcorn and toss until well coated.
Season popcorn with salt and black pepper, toss until mixed and serve.

Masala Popcorn

Total time: 20 minutes
Ingredients
3 cups popped popcorn
2 hot chili peppers, sliced
1 teaspoon ground cumin
6 curry leaves
1 teaspoon ground coriander
1/3 teaspoon salt
1/8 teaspoon chaat masala
1/4 teaspoon turmeric powder
¼ teaspoon red pepper flakes
1/4 teaspoon garam masala
1/3 cup olive oil
Directions:
Take a large pot, place it over medium heat, add half of the oil and when hot, add chili peppers and curry leaves and cook for 3 minutes until golden.
When done, transfer curry leaves and pepper to a plate lined with paper towels and set aside until required.
Add remaining oil into the pot, add remaining ingredients except for popcorns, stir until mixed and cook for 1 minute until fragrant.
Then tip in popcorns, remove the pan from heat, stir well until coated, and then sprinkle with bay leaves and red chili.
Toss until mixed and serve straight away.

Applesauce

Total time: 25 minutes
Ingredients
4 pounds mixed apples, cored, ½-inch chopped
1 strip of orange peel, about 3-inch
1/2 cup coconut sugar
1/2 teaspoon salt
1 cinnamon stick, about 3-inch
2 tablespoons apple cider vinegar
Apple cider as needed for consistency of the sauce
Directions:
Take a large pot, place apples in it, then add remaining ingredients except for cider, stir until mixed and cook for 15 minutes over medium heat until apples have wilted, stirring every 10 minutes.
When done, remove the cinnamon stick and orange peel and puree the mixture by using an immersion blender until smooth and stir in apple cider until sauce reaches to desired consistency.
Serve straight away.

Black Bean and Corn Quesadillas

Total time: 45 minutes
Ingredients
For the Black Beans and Corn:
1/2 of a medium white onion, peeled, chopped
1/2 cup cooked black beans
1/2 cup cooked corn kernels
1 teaspoon minced garlic
½ of jalapeno, deseeded, diced
1/2 teaspoon salt
1 teaspoon red chili powder
1 teaspoon cumin
1 tablespoon olive oil
For the Quesadillas:
4 large corn tortillas
4 green onions, chopped
½ cup vegan nacho cheese sauce
½ cup chopped cilantro
1 large tomato, diced
Salsa as needed for dipping
Directions:
Prepare beans and for this, take a frying pan, place it over medium-high heat, add oil and when hot, add onion, jalapeno, and garlic and cook for 3 minutes.
Then add remaining ingredients, stir until mixed and cook for 2 minutes until hot.
Take a large skillet pan, place over medium heat, place the tortilla in it and cook for 1 minute until toasted and then flip it.
Spread some of the cheese sauce on one half of the top, spread with beans mixture, top with cilantro, onion, and tomato and then fold the filling with the other side of the tortilla.
Pat down the tortilla, cook it for 2 minutes, then carefully flip it, continue cooking for 2 minutes until hot, and then slide to a plate.
Cook remaining quesadilla in the same manner, then cut them into wedges and serve.

Zaatar Popcorn

Total time: 10 minutes
Ingredients
8 cups popped popcorns
1/4 cup za'atar spice blend
¾ teaspoon salt
4 tablespoons olive oil
Directions:
Place all the ingredients except for popcorns in a large bowl and whisk until combined.
Then add popcorns, toss until well coated, and serve straight away.

Chocolate-Covered Almonds

Total time: 1 hour 45 minutes 30 seconds
Ingredients
8 ounces almonds
1/2 teaspoon sea salt
6 ounces chocolate disks, semisweet, melted
Directions:
Microwave chocolate in a heatproof bowl for 30 seconds until it melts, then dip almonds in it, four at a time, and place them on a baking sheet.
Let almonds stand for 1 hour until hardened, then sprinkle with salt, and cool them in the refrigerator for 30 minutes.
Serve straight away.

Beans and Spinach Tacos

Total time: 25 minutes
Ingredients
12 ounces spinach
4 tablespoons cooked kidney beans
½ of medium red onion, peeled, chopped
½ teaspoon minced garlic
1 medium tomato, chopped
3 tablespoons chopped parsley
½ of avocado, sliced
½ teaspoon ground black pepper
1 teaspoon salt
2 tablespoons olive oil
4 slices of vegan brie cheese
4 tortillas, about 6-inches
Directions:
Take a skillet pan, place it over medium heat, add oil and when hot, add onion and cook for 10 minutes until softened.
Then stir in spinach, cook for 4 minutes until its leaves wilts, then drain it and distribute evenly between tortillas.
Top evenly with remaining ingredients, season with black pepper and salt, drizzle with lemon juice and then serve.

Zucchini and Amaranth Patties

Total time: 40 minutes
Ingredients
1 1/2 cups shredded zucchini
½ of a medium onion, shredded
1 1/2 cups cooked white beans
1/2 cup amaranth seeds
1 teaspoon red chili powder
1/2 teaspoon cumin
1/2 cup cornmeal
1/4 cup flax meal
1 tablespoon salsa
1 1/2 cups vegetable broth
Directions:
Stir together stock and amaranth on a pot, bring it to a boil over medium-high heat, then switch heat to medium-low level and simmer until all the liquid is absorbed.
Mash the white beans in a bowl, add remaining ingredients including cooked amaranth and stir until well mixed.
Shape the mixture into patties, then place them on a baking sheet lined with parchment sheet and bake for 30 minutes until browned and crispy, turning halfway.
Serve straight away.

Rice Pizza

Total time: 45 minutes
Ingredients
For the Crust:
1 1/2 cup short-grain rice, cooked
1/2 teaspoon garlic powder
1 teaspoon coconut sugar
1 tablespoon red chili flakes
For the Sauce:
1/4 teaspoon onion powder
1 tablespoon nutritional yeast
1/4 teaspoon garlic powder
1/4 teaspoon ginger powder
1 tablespoon red chili flakes
1 teaspoon soy sauce
1/2 cup tomato purée
For the Toppings:
2 1/2 cups oyster mushrooms
1 chili pepper, deseeded, sliced
2 scallions, sliced
1 teaspoon coconut sugar
1 teaspoon soy sauce
Baby corn as needed
Directions:
Prepare the crust and for this, place all of its ingredients in a bowl and stir until well combined.
Then take a pizza pan, line it with parchment sheet, place rice mixture in it, spread it evenly, and then bake for 20 minutes at 350 degrees F.
Then spread tomato sauce over the crust, top evenly with remaining ingredients for the topping and continue baking for 15 minutes.
When done, slice the pizza into wedges and serve.

Loaded Baked Potatoes

Total time: 42 minutes
Ingredients
1/2 cup cooked chickpeas
2 medium potatoes, scrubbed
1 cup broccoli florets, steamed
1/4 cup vegan bacon bits
2 tablespoons all-purpose seasoning
¼ cup vegan cheese sauce
1/2 cup vegan sour cream
Directions:
Pierce hole in the potatoes, microwave them for 12 minutes over high heat setting until soft to touch, and then bake them for 20 minutes at 450 degrees F until very tender.
Open the potatoes, mash the flesh with a fork, then top evenly with remaining ingredients and serve.

Coconut Rice

Total time: 25 minutes
Ingredients
1 1/2 cups white rice
1 teaspoon coconut sugar
1/8 teaspoon salt
14 ounces coconut milk, unsweetened
1 1/4 cups water
Directions:
Take a saucepan, place it over medium heat, add all the ingredients in it, stir well and bring the mixture to a boil.
Switch heat to medium-low level, simmer the rice for 20 minutes until tender, and then serve straight away.

Potato Chips

Total time: 30 minutes
Ingredients
3 medium potatoes, scrubbed, thinly sliced, soaked in warm water for 10 min
½ teaspoon garlic powder
½ teaspoon onion powder
½ teaspoon red chili powder
½ teaspoon curry powder
1 teaspoon of sea salt
1 tablespoon apple cider vinegar
2 tablespoons olive oil
Directions:
Drain the potato slices, pat dry, then place them in a large bowl, add remaining ingredients and toss until well coated.
Spread the potatoes in a single layer on a baking sheet and bake for 20 minutes until crispy, turning halfway.
Serve straight away.

Spinach and Artichoke Dip

Total time: 35 minutes
Ingredients
28 ounces artichokes
1 small white onion, peeled, diced
1 1/2 cups cashews, soaked, drained
4 cups spinach
4 cloves of garlic, peeled
1 1 1/2 teaspoons salt
1/4 cup nutritional yeast
1 tablespoon olive oil
2 tablespoons lemon juice
1 1/2 cups coconut milk, unsweetened
Directions:
Cook onion and garlic in hot oil for 3 minutes until saute and then set aside until required.
Place cashews in a food processor; add 1 teaspoon salt, yeast, milk, and lemon juice and pulse until smooth.
Add spinach, onion mixture, and artichokes and pulse until the chunky mixture comes together.
Tip the dip in a heatproof dish and bake for 20 minutes at 425 degrees F until the top is browned and dip bubbles.
Serve straight away with vegetable sticks.

Avocado Toast with Herbs and Peas

Total time: 10 minutes
Ingredients
½ of a medium avocado, peeled, pitted, mashed
6 slices of radish
2 tablespoons baby peas
¼ teaspoon ground black pepper
1 teaspoon chopped basil
¼ teaspoon salt
1/2 lemon, juiced
1 slice of bread, whole-grain, toasted
Directions:
Spread mashed avocado on the one side of the toast and then top with peas, pressing them into the avocado.
Layer the toast with radish slices, season with salt and black pepper, sprinkle with basil, and drizzle with lemon juice.
Serve straight away.

Oven-Dried Grapes

Total time: 4 hours 5 minutes
Ingredients
3 large bunches of grapes, seedless
Olive oil as needed for greasing
Directions:
Spread grapes into two greased baking sheets and bake for 4 hours at 225 degrees F until semi-dried.
When done, let the grape cool completely and then serve.

Queso Dip

Total time: 5 minutes
 Ingredients
1 cup cashews
½ teaspoon minced garlic
1/2 teaspoon salt
1/2 teaspoon ground cumin
1 teaspoon red chili powder
2 tablespoons nutritional yeast
1 tablespoon harissa
1 cup hot water
Directions:
Place all the ingredients in a food processor and pulse for 2 minutes until smooth and well combined.
Tip the dip in a bowl, taste to adjust seasoning and then serve.

Nooch Popcorn

Total time: 20 minutes
 Ingredients
1/3 cup nutritional yeast
1 teaspoon of sea salt
3 tablespoons coconut oil
½ cup popcorn kernels
Directions:
Place yeast in a large bowl, stir in salt, and set aside until required.
Take a medium saucepan, place it over medium-high heat, add oil and when it melts, add four kernels and wait until they sizzle.
Then add remaining kernel, toss until coated, shut the pan with the lid, and shake the kernels until popped completely.
When done, transfer popcorns tot eh yeast mixture, shut with lid and shape well until coated.
Serve straight away

Honey-Almond Popcorn

Total time: 15 minutes
Ingredients
1/2 cup popcorn kernels
2 tablespoons honey
1/2 teaspoon sea salt
2 tablespoons coconut sugar
1 cup roasted almonds
1/4 cup walnut oil
Directions:
Take a pot, place it over medium-low heat, add oil and when it melts, add four kernels and wait until they sizzle.
Then add remaining kernel, toss until coated, sprinkle with sugar, drizzle with honey, shut the pot with the lid, and shake the kernels until popped completely, adding almonds halfway.
Once all the kernels have popped, season them with salt and serve straight away.

Turmeric Snack Bites

Total time: 35 minutes
Ingredients
1 cup Medjool dates, pitted, chopped
1/2 cup walnuts
1 teaspoon ground turmeric
1 tablespoon cocoa powder, unsweetened
1/2 teaspoon cinnamon
1/2 cup shredded coconut, unsweetened
Directions:
Place all the ingredients in a food processor and pulse for 2 minutes until a smooth mixture comes together.
Tip the mixture in a bowl and then shape it into ten small balls, 1 tablespoon of the mixture per ball and then refrigerate for 30 minutes.
Serve straight away.

Avocado Tomato Bruschetta

Total time: 10 minutes
Ingredients
3 slices of whole-grain bread
6 chopped cherry tomatoes
½ of sliced avocado
½ teaspoon minced garlic
½ teaspoon ground black pepper
2 tablespoons chopped basil
½ teaspoon of sea salt
1 teaspoon balsamic vinegar
Directions:
Place tomatoes in a bowl, and then stir in vinegar until mixed.
Top bread slices with avocado slices, then top evenly with tomato mixture, garlic and basil, and season with salt and black pepper.
Serve straight away

Cinnamon Bananas

Total time: 13 minutes
Ingredients
2 bananas, peeled, sliced
1 teaspoon cinnamon
2 tablespoons granulated Splenda
1/4 teaspoon nutmeg
Directions
Prepare the cinnamon mixture and for this, place all the ingredients in a bowl, except for banana, and stir until mixed.
Take a large skillet pan, place it over medium heat, spray with oil, add banana slices and sprinkle with half of the prepared cinnamon mixture.
Cook for 3 minutes, then sprinkle with remaining prepared cinnamon mixture and continue cooking for 3 minutes until tender and hot.
Serve straight away.

Red Salsa

Total time: 10 minutes
Ingredients
30 ounces diced fire-roasted tomatoes
4 tablespoons diced green chilies
1 medium jalapeño pepper, deseeded
1/2 cup chopped green onion
1 cup chopped cilantro
1 teaspoon minced garlic
½ teaspoon of sea salt
1 teaspoon ground cumin
¼ teaspoon stevia
3 tablespoons lime juice
Directions:
Place all the ingredients in a food processor and process for 2 minutes until smooth.
Tip the salsa in a bowl, taste to adjust seasoning and then serve.

Tomato Hummus

Total time: 5 minutes
Ingredients
1/4 cup sun-dried tomatoes, without oil
1 ½ cups cooked chickpeas
1 teaspoon minced garlic
1/2 teaspoon salt
2 tablespoons sesame oil
1 tablespoon lemon juice
1 tablespoon olive oil
1/4 cup of water
Directions:
Place all the ingredients in a food processor and process for 2 minutes until smooth.
Tip the hummus in a bowl, drizzle with more oil, and then serve straight away.

Zucchini Chips

Total time: 130 minutes
Ingredients
1 large zucchini, thinly sliced
1 teaspoon salt
2 tablespoons olive oil
Directions:
Pat dry zucchini slices and then spread them in an even layer on a baking sheet lined with parchment sheet.
Whisk together salt and oil, brush this mixture over zucchini slices on both sides and then bake for 2 hours or more until brown and crispy.
When done, let the chips cool for 10 minutes and then serve straight away.

Rosemary Beet Chips

Total time: 30 minutes
Ingredients
3 large beets, scrubbed, thinly sliced
1/8 teaspoon ground black pepper
¼ teaspoon of sea salt
3 sprigs of rosemary, leaves chopped
4 tablespoons olive oil
Directions:
Spread beet slices in a single layer between two large baking sheets, brush the slices with oil, then season with spices and rosemary, toss until well coated, and bake for 20 minutes at 375 degrees F until crispy, turning halfway.
When done, let the chips cool for 10 minutes and then serve.

Tomato and Pesto Toast

Total time: 5 minutes
 Ingredients
1 small tomato, sliced
¼ teaspoon ground black pepper
1 tablespoon vegan pesto
2 tablespoons hummus
1 slice of whole-grain bread, toasted
Hemp seeds as needed for garnishing
Directions:
Spread hummus on one side of the toast, top with tomato slices and then drizzle with pesto.
Sprinkle black pepper on the toast along with hemp seeds and then serve straight away.

Avocado and Sprout Toast

Total time: 5 minutes
Ingredients
1/2 of a medium avocado, sliced
1 slice of whole-grain bread, toasted
2 tablespoons sprouts
2 tablespoons hummus
¼ teaspoon lemon zest
½ teaspoon hemp seeds
¼ teaspoon red pepper flakes
Directions:
Spread hummus on one side of the toast and then top with avocado slices and sprouts.
Sprinkle with lemon zest, hemp seeds, and red pepper flakes and then serve straight away.

Zucchini Hummus

Total time: 5 minutes
 Ingredients
1 cup diced zucchini
1/2 teaspoon sea salt
1 teaspoon minced garlic
2 teaspoons ground cumin
3 tablespoons lemon juice
1/3 cup tahini
Directions:
Place all the ingredients in a food processor and pulse for 2 minutes until smooth.
Tip the hummus in a bowl, drizzle with oil and serve.

Chipotle and Lime Tortilla Chips

Total time: 25 minutes
Ingredients
12 ounces whole-wheat tortillas
4 tablespoons chipotle seasoning
1 tablespoon olive oil
4 limes, juiced
Directions:
Whisk together oil and lime juice, brush it well on tortillas, then sprinkle with chipotle seasoning and bake for 15 minutes at 350 degrees F until crispy, turning halfway.
When done, let the tortilla cool for 10 minutes, then break it into chips and serve.

Chapter 9: Desserts Recipes

Peanut Butter Energy Bars

Total time: 5 hours 20 minutes
Ingredients
1/2 cup cranberries
12 Medjool dates, pitted
1 cup roasted almond
1 tablespoon chia seeds
1 1/2 cups oats
1/8 teaspoon salt
1/4 cup and 1 tablespoon agave nectar
1/2 teaspoon vanilla extract, unsweetened
1/3 cup and 1 tablespoon peanut butter, unsalted
2 tablespoons water
Directions:
Place an almond in a food processor, pulse until chopped, and then transfer into a large bowl.
Add dates into the food processor along with oats, pour in water, and pulse for dates are chopped.
Add dates mixture into the almond mixture, add chia seeds and berries and stir until mixed.
Take a saucepan, place it over medium heat, add remaining butter and remaining ingredients, stir and cook for 5 minutes until mixture reaches to a liquid consistency.
Pour the butter mixture over date mixture, and then stir until well combined.
Take an 8 by 8 inches baking tray, line it with parchment sheet, add date mixture in it, spread and press it evenly and refrigerate for 5 hours.
Cut it into sixteen bars and serve.

Black Bean Brownie Pops

Total time: 47 minutes
Ingredients
3/4 cup chocolate chips
15 ounce cooked black beans
1 tablespoon maple syrup
5 tablespoons cacao powder
1/8 teaspoon sea salt
2 tablespoons sunflower seed butter
Directions:
Place black beans in a food processor, add remaining ingredients, except for chocolate, and pulse for 2 minutes until combined and the dough starts to come together.
Shape the dough into twelve balls, arrange them on a baking sheet lined with parchment paper, then insert a toothpick into each ball and refrigerate for 20 minutes.
Then meat chocolate in the microwave for 2 minutes, and dip brownie pops in it until covered.
Return the pops into the refrigerator for 10 minutes until set and then serve.

Caramel Brownie Slice

Total time: 4 hours
Ingredients
For the Base:
¼ cup dried figs
½ cup cacao powder
½ cup pecans
½ cup walnuts
For the Caramel Layer:
¼ teaspoons sea salt
3 Tablespoons coconut oil
5 Tablespoons water
For the Chocolate Topping:
1/3 cup agave nectar
½ cup cacao powder
¼ cup of coconut oil
1 cup dried dates
Directions:
Prepare the base, and for this, place all its ingredients in a food processor and pulse for 3 to 5 minutes until the thick paste comes together.
Take an 8 by 8 inches baking dish, grease it with oil, place base mixture in it and spread and press the mixture evenly in the bottom, and freeze until required.
Prepare the caramel layer, and for this, place all its ingredients in a food processor and pulse for 2 minutes until smooth.
Pour the caramel into the prepared baking dish, smooth the top and freeze for 20 minutes.
Then prepare the topping and for this, place all its ingredients in a food processor, and pulse for 1 minute until combined.
Gently spread the chocolate mixture over the caramel layer and then freeze for 3 hours until set.
Serve straight away.

Snickers Pie

Total time: 4 hours
Ingredients
For the Crust:
12 Medjool dates, pitted
1 cup dried coconut, unsweetened
5 tablespoons cocoa powder
1/2 teaspoon sea salt
1 teaspoon vanilla extract, unsweetened
1 cup almonds
For the Caramel Layer:
10 Medjool dates, pitted, soaked for 10 minutes in warm water, drained
3 teaspoons vanilla extract, unsweetened
3 teaspoons coconut oil
3 tablespoons almond butter, unsalted
For the Peanut Butter Mousse:
3/4 cup peanut butter
2 tablespoons maple syrup
1/2 teaspoon vanilla extract, unsweetened
1/8 teaspoon sea salt
28 ounces coconut milk, chilled
Directions:
Prepare the crust, and for this, place all its ingredients in a food processor and pulse for 3 to 5 minutes until the thick paste comes together.
Take a baking pan, line it with parchment paper, place crust mixture in it and spread and press the mixture evenly in the bottom, and freeze until required.
Prepare the caramel layer, and for this, place all its ingredients in a food processor and pulse for 2 minutes until smooth.
Pour the caramel on top of the prepared crust, smooth the top and freeze for 30 minutes until set.
Prepare the mousse and for this, separate coconut milk and its solid, then add solid from coconut milk into a food processor, add remaining ingredients and then pulse for 1 minute until smooth.
Top prepared mousse over caramel layer, and then freeze for 3 hours until set.
Serve straight away.

Matcha Coconut Cream Pie

Total time: 5 minutes

Ingredients

For the Crust:

1/2 cup ground flaxseed

3/4 cup shredded dried coconut

1 cup Medjool dates, pitted

3/4 cup dehydrated buckwheat groats

1/4 teaspoons sea salt

For the Filling:

1 cup dried coconut flakes

4 cups of coconut meat

1/4 cup and 2 Tablespoons coconut nectar

1/2 Tablespoons vanilla extract, unsweetened

1/4 teaspoons sea salt

2/3 cup and 2 Tablespoons coconut butter

1 Tablespoons matcha powder

1/2 cup coconut water

Directions:

Prepare the crust, and for this, place all its ingredients in a food processor and pulse for 3 to 5 minutes until the thick paste comes together.

Take a 6-inch springform pan, grease it with oil, place crust mixture in it and spread and press the mixture evenly in the bottom and along the sides, and freeze until required.

Prepare the filling and for this, place all its ingredients in a food processor, and pulse for 2 minutes until smooth.

Pour the filling into prepared pan, smooth the top, and freeze for 4 hours until set.

Cut pie into slices and then serve.

Chocolate Peanut Butter Cake

Total time: 5 minutes
Ingredients
For the Base:
1 tablespoon ground flaxseeds
1/8 cup millet
3/4 cup peanuts
1/4 cup and 2 tablespoons shredded coconut unsweetened
1 teaspoon hemp oil
1/2 cup flake oats
For the Date Layer:
1 tablespoon ground flaxseed
1 cup dates
1 tablespoon hemp hearts
2 tablespoons coconut
3 tablespoons cacao
For the Chocolate Layer:
3/4 cup coconut flour
2 tablespoons and 2 teaspoons cacao
1 tablespoon maple syrup
8 tablespoons warm water
2 tablespoons coconut oil
1/2 cup coconut milk
2 tablespoons ground flaxseed
For the Chocolate Topping:
7 ounces coconut cream
2 1/2 tablespoons cacao
1 teaspoon agave
For Assembly:
1/2 cup almond butter
Directions:
Prepare the crust, and for this, place all its ingredients in a food processor and pulse for 3 to 5 minutes until the thick paste comes together.
Take a loaf tin, grease it with oil, place crust mixture in it and spread and press the mixture evenly in the bottom and along the sides, and freeze until required.
Prepare the date layer, and for this, place all its ingredients in a food processor and pulse for 2 minutes until smooth.
Prepare the chocolate layer, and for this, place flour and flax in a bowl and stir until combined.
Take a saucepan, add remaining ingredients, stir until mixed and cook for 5 minutes until melted and smooth.
Add it into the flour mixture, stir until dough comes together, and set aside.
Prepare the chocolate topping, place all its ingredients in a food processor and pulse for 3 to 5 minutes until smooth.
Press date layer into the base layer, refrigerate for 1 hour, then press chocolate layer on its top, finish with chocolate topping, refrigerate for 3 hours and serve.

Strawberry Mousse

Total time: 20 minutes
Ingredients
8 ounces coconut milk, unsweetened
2 tablespoons honey
5 strawberries
Directions:
Place berries in a blender and pulse until the smooth mixture comes together.
Place milk in a bowl, whisk until whipped, and then add remaining ingredients and stir until combined.
Refrigerate the mousse for 10 minutes and then serve.

Blueberry Mousse

Total time: 20 minutes
Ingredients
1 cup wild blueberries
1 cup cashews, soaked for 10 minutes, drained
1/2 teaspoon berry powder
2 tablespoons coconut oil, melted
1 tablespoon lemon juice
1 teaspoon vanilla extract, unsweetened
1/4 cup hot water
Directions:
Place all the ingredients in a food processor and process for 2 minutes until smooth.
Set aside until required.

Chocolate Raspberry Brownies

Total time: 4 hours
Ingredients
For the Chocolate Brownie Base:
12 Medjool Dates, pitted
3/4 cup oat flour
3/4 cup almond meal
3 tablespoons cacao
1 teaspoon vanilla extract, unsweetened
1/8 teaspoon sea salt
3 tablespoons water
1/2 cup pecans, chopped
For the Raspberry Cheesecake:
3/4 cup cashews, soaked, drained
6 tablespoons agave nectar
1/2 cup raspberries
1 teaspoon vanilla extract, unsweetened
1 lemon, juiced
6 tablespoons liquid coconut oil
For the Chocolate Coating:
2 1/2 tablespoons cacao powder
3 3/4 tablespoons coconut Oil
2 tablespoons maple syrup
1/8 teaspoon sea salt
Directions:
Prepare the crust, and for this, place all its ingredients in a food processor and pulse for 3 to 5 minutes until the thick paste comes together.
Take a 6-inch springform pan, grease it with oil, place crust mixture in it and spread and press the mixture evenly in the bottom and along the sides, and freeze until required.
Prepare the cheesecake topping, and for this, place all its ingredients in a food processor and pulse for 2 minutes until smooth.
Pour the filling into prepared pan, smooth the top, and freeze for 8 hours until solid.
Prepare the chocolate coating and for this, whisk together all its ingredients until smooth, drizzle on top of the cake and then serve.

Brownie Batter

Total time: 5 minutes
Ingredients
4 Medjool dates, pitted, soaked in warm water
1.5 ounces chocolate, unsweetened, melted
2 tablespoons maple syrup
4 tablespoons tahini
½ teaspoon vanilla extract, unsweetened
1 tablespoon cocoa powder, unsweetened
1/8 teaspoon sea salt
1/8 teaspoon espresso powder
2 to 4 tablespoons almond milk, unsweetened
Directions:
Place all the ingredients in a food processor and process for 2 minutes until combined.
Set aside until required.

Double Chocolate Orange Cheesecake

Total time: 4 hours
Ingredients
For the Base:
9 Medjool dates, pitted
1/3 cup Brazil nuts
2 tablespoons maple syrup
1/3 cup walnuts
2 tablespoons water
3 tablespoons cacao powder
For the Chocolate Cheesecake:
1/2 cup cacao powder
1 1/2 cups cashews, soaked for 10 minutes in warm water, drained
1/3 cup liquid coconut oil
1 teaspoon vanilla extract, unsweetened
1/3 cup maple syrup
1/3 cup water
For the Orange Cheesecake:
2 oranges, juiced
1/4 cup maple syrup
1 cup cashews, soaked for 10 minutes in warm water, drained
1 teaspoon vanilla extract, unsweetened
2 tablespoons coconut butter
1/2 cup liquid coconut oil
2 oranges, zested
4 drops of orange essential oil
For the Chocolate Topping:
3 tablespoons cacao powder
3 drops of orange essential oil
2 tablespoons liquid coconut oil
3 tablespoons maple syrup
Directions:
Prepare the base, and for this, place all its ingredients in a food processor and pulse for 3 to 5 minutes until the thick paste comes together.
Take a cake tin, place crust mixture in it and spread and press the mixture evenly in the bottom, and freeze until required.
Prepare the chocolate cheesecake, and for this, place all its ingredients in a food processor and pulse for 2 minutes until smooth.
Pour the chocolate cheesecake mixture on top of the prepared base, smooth the top and freeze for 20 minutes until set.
Then prepare the orange cheesecake and for this, place all its ingredients in a food processor, and pulse for 2 minutes until smooth
Top orange cheesecake mixture over chocolate cheesecake, and then freeze for 3 hours until hardened.
Then prepare the chocolate topping and for this, take a bowl, add all the ingredients in it and stir until well combined.
Spread chocolate topping over the top, freeze the cake for 10 minutes until the topping has hardened and then slice to serve.

Coconut Ice Cream Cheesecake

Total time: 3 hours
Ingredients
For the First Layer:
1 cup mixed nuts
3/4 cup dates, soaked for 10 minutes in warm water
2 tablespoons almond milk
For the Second Layer:
1 medium avocado, diced
1 cup cashew nuts, soaked for 10 minutes in warm water
3 cups strawberries, sliced
1 tablespoon chia seeds, soaked in 3 tablespoons soy milk
1/2 cup agave
1 cup melted coconut oil
1/2 cup shredded coconut
1 lime, juiced
Directions:
Prepare the first layer, and for this, place all its ingredients in a food processor and pulse for 3 to 5 minutes until the thick paste comes together.
Take a springform pan, place crust mixture in it and spread and press the mixture evenly in the bottom, and freeze until required.
Prepare the second layer, and for this, place all its ingredients in a food processor and pulse for 2 minutes until smooth.
Pour the second layer on top of the first layer, smooth the top, and freeze for 4 hours until hard.
Serve straight away.

Lemon Cashew Tart

Total time: 3 hours 15 minutes
Ingredients
For the Crust:
1 cup almonds
4 dates, pitted, soaked in warm water for 10 minutes in water, drained
1/8 teaspoon crystal salt
1 teaspoon vanilla extract, unsweetened
For the Cream:
1 cup cashews, soaked in warm water for 10 minutes in water, drained
1/4 cup water
1/4 cup coconut nectar
1 teaspoon coconut oil
1 teaspoon vanilla extract, unsweetened
1 lemon, Juiced
1/8 teaspoon crystal salt
For the Topping:
Shredded coconut as needed
Directions:
Prepare the cream and for this, place all its ingredients in a food processor, pulse for 2 minutes until smooth, and then refrigerate for 1 hour.
Then prepare the crust, and for this, place all its ingredients in a food processor and pulse for 3 to 5 minutes until the thick paste comes together.
Take a tart pan, grease it with oil, place crust mixture in it and spread and press the mixture evenly in the bottom and along the sides, and freeze until required.
Pour the filling into the prepared tart, smooth the top, and refrigerate for 2 hours until set.
Cut tart into slices and then serve.

Peppermint Oreos

Total time: 2 hours
Ingredients
For the Cookies:
1 cup dates
2/3 cup brazil nuts
3 tablespoons carob powder
2/3 cup almonds
1/8 teaspoon sea salt
3 tablespoons water
For the Crème:
2 tablespoons almond butter
1 cup coconut chips
2 tablespoons melted coconut oil
1 cup coconut shreds
3 drops of peppermint oil
1/2 teaspoon vanilla powder
For the Dark Chocolate:
3/4 cup cacao powder
1/2 cup date paste
1/3 cup coconut oil, melted

Directions:
Prepare the cookies, and for this, place all its ingredients in a food processor and pulse for 3 to 5 minutes until the dough comes together.
Then place the dough between two parchment sheets, roll the dough, then cut out twenty-four cookies of the desired shape and freeze until solid.
Prepare the crème, and for this, place all its ingredients in a food processor and pulse for 2 minutes until smooth. When cookies have harden, sandwich crème in between the cookies by placing dollops on top of a cookie and then pressing it with another cookie.
Freeze the cookies for 30 minutes and in the meantime, prepare chocolate and for this, place all its ingredients in a bowl and whisk until combined.
Dip frouncesen cookie sandwich into chocolate, at least two times, and then freeze for another 30 minutes until chocolate has hardened.
Serve straight away.

Key Lime Pie

Total time: 3 hours 15 minutes
Ingredients
For the Crust:
¾ cup coconut flakes, unsweetened
1 cup dates, soaked in warm water for 10 minutes in water, drained
For the Filling:
¾ cup of coconut meat
1 ½ avocado, peeled, pitted
2 tablespoons key lime juice
¼ cup agave

Directions:
Prepare the crust, and for this, place all its ingredients in a food processor and pulse for 3 to 5 minutes until the thick paste comes together.
Take an 8-inch pie pan, grease it with oil, pour crust mixture in it and spread and press the mixture evenly in the bottom and along the sides, and freeze until required.
Prepare the filling and for this, place all its ingredients in a food processor, and pulse for 2 minutes until smooth. Pour the filling into prepared pan, smooth the top, and freeze for 3 hours until set.
Cut pie into slices and then serve.

Chocolate Mint Grasshopper Pie

Total time: 4 hours 15 minutes
Ingredients
For the Crust:
1 cup dates, soaked in warm water for 10 minutes in water, drained
1/8 teaspoons salt
1/2 cup pecans
1 teaspoons cinnamon
1/2 cup walnuts
For the Filling:
½ cup mint leaves
2 cups of cashews, soaked in warm water for 10 minutes in water, drained
2 tablespoons coconut oil
1/4 cup and 2 tablespoons of agave
1/4 teaspoons spirulina
1/4 cup water
Directions:
Prepare the crust, and for this, place all its ingredients in a food processor and pulse for 3 to 5 minutes until the thick paste comes together.
Take a 6-inch springform pan, grease it with oil, place crust mixture in it and spread and press the mixture evenly in the bottom and along the sides, and freeze until required.
Prepare the filling and for this, place all its ingredients in a food processor, and pulse for 2 minutes until smooth.
Pour the filling into prepared pan, smooth the top, and freeze for 4 hours until set.
Cut pie into slices and then serve.

Oatmeal Raisin Muffins

Total time: 45 minutes
Ingredients
2½ cups rolled oats
½ cup oat flour
1 teaspoon baking powder
½ teaspoon baking soda
1 teaspoon salt
1 tablespoon cinnamon
½ teaspoon ground nutmeg
4 ripe bananas, mashed
1 apple, grated
½ cup almond milk
3 teaspoons vanilla extract
½ cup raisins
½ cup chopped walnuts
Directions:
Preheat your oven to 350 degrees F.
Whisk the dry ingredients in a mixing bowl, and wet ingredients in a separate bowl.
Beat the two mixtures together until smooth.
Fold in apples, walnuts and raisins, give it a gentle stir.
Line a muffin tray with muffin cups and evenly divide the muffin batter among the cups.
Bake for nearly 35 minutes and serve.

Fudge Popsicles

Total time: 2 hours 10 minutes
Ingredients
1 cup almond milk
3 ripe bananas
3 tablespoon cocoa powder
1 tablespoon almond butter
Directions:
In a blender, blend all the ingredients for popsicles until smooth.
Divide the popsicle blend into the popsicle molds.
Insert the popsicles sticks and close the molds.
Place the molds in the freezer for 2 hours to set.
Serve.

Strawberry Coconut Popsicles

Total time: 2 hours 10 minutes
Ingredients
2 medium bananas, sliced
1 can coconut milk
1 cup strawberries
3 tablespoons maple syrup
Directions:
In a blender, blend all the ingredients for popsicles until smooth.
Divide the popsicle blend into the popsicle molds.
Insert the popsicles sticks and close the molds.
Place the molds in the freezer for 2 hours to set.
Serve.

Green Popsicle

Total time: hours 10 minutes
Ingredients
1 ripe avocado, peeled and pitted
1 cup fresh spinach
1 can (13.5 ounce) full fat coconut milk
¼ cup lime juice
2 tablespoons maple syrup
1 teaspoon vanilla extract
Directions:
In a blender, blend all the ingredients for popsicles until smooth.
Divide the popsicle blend into the popsicle molds.
Insert the popsicles sticks and close the molds.
Place the molds in the freezer for 2 hours to set.
Serve.

Peach Popsicles

Total time: 2 hours 10 minutes
Ingredients
2½ cups peaches, peeled and pitted
2 tablespoons agave
¾ cup coconut cream
Directions:
In a blender, blend all the ingredients for popsicles until smooth.
Divide the popsicle blend into the popsicle molds.
Insert the popsicles sticks and close the molds.
Place the molds in the freezer for 2 hours to set.
Serve.

Coconut Fat Bombs

Total time: 1 hour 11 minutes
Ingredients
1 can coconut milk
¾ cup coconut oil
1 cup coconut flakes
20 drops liquid stevia
Directions:
In a bowl combine all the ingredients.
Melt in a microwave for 1 minute.
Mix well then divide the mixture into silicone molds.
Freeze them for 1 hour to set.
Serve.

Apple Pie Bites

Total time: 1 hour 10 minutes
Ingredients
1 cup walnuts, chopped
½ cup coconut oil
¼ cup ground flax seeds
½ ounce freeze dried apples
1 teaspoon vanilla extract
1 teaspoon cinnamon
Liquid stevia, to taste
Directions:
In a bowl add all the ingredients.
Mix well then roll the mixture into small balls.
Freeze them for 1 hour to set.
Serve.

Mojito Fat Bombs

Total time: 1 hour 11 minutes
Ingredients
¾ cup hulled hemp seeds
½ cup coconut oil
1 cup fresh mint
½ teaspoon mint extract
Juice & zest of two limes
¼ teaspoon stevia
Directions:
In a bowl, combine all the ingredients.
Melt in the microwave for 1 minute.
Mix well then divide the mixture into silicone molds.
Freeze them for 1 hour to set.
Serve.

Protein Fat Bombs

Total time: 1 hour 10 minutes
Ingredients
1 cup coconut oil
1 cup peanut butter, melted
½ cup cocoa powder
¼ cup plant-based protein powder
1 pinch of salt
2 cups unsweetened shredded coconut
Directions:
In a bowl, add all the ingredients except coconut shreds.
Mix well then make small balls out of this mixture and place them into silicone molds.
Freeze for 1 hour to set.
Roll the balls in the coconut shreds
Serve.

Chocolate Peanut Fat Bombs

Total time: 1 hour 11 minutes
Ingredients
½ cup coconut butter
1 cup plus 2 tablespoons peanut butter
5 tablespoons cocoa powder
2 teaspoons maple syrup
Directions:
In a bowl, combine all the ingredients.
Melt them in the microwave for 1 minute.
Mix well then divide the mixture into silicone molds.
Freeze them for 1 hour to set.
Serve.

Carrot Flaxseed Muffins

Total time: 30 minutes
Ingredients
2 tablespoons ground flax
5 tablespoons water
¾ cup almond milk
¾ cup applesauce
½ cup maple syrup
1 teaspoon vanilla extract
1½ cups whole wheat flour
½ cup rolled oats
1 teaspoon baking soda
1½ teaspoon baking powder
¼ teaspoon ground ginger
1 teaspoon salt
1 teaspoon cinnamon
1 cup grated carrot
Directions:
Whisk flaxseed with water in a bowl and leave it for 10 minutes
Preheat your oven to 350 degrees F.
Separately, whisk together the dry ingredients in one bowl and the wet ingredients in another bowl.
Beat the two mixtures together until smooth.
Fold in flaxseed and carrots, give it a gentle stir.
Line a muffin tray with muffin cups and evenly divide the muffin batter among the cups.
Bake for 20 minutes and serve.

Banana Walnut Muffins

Total time: 28 minutes
Ingredients
4 large pitted dates, boiled
1 cup almond milk
2 tablespoons lemon juice
2½ cups rolled oats
1 teaspoon baking powder
1 teaspoon baking soda
1 teaspoon cinnamon
¼ teaspoon nutmeg
⅛ teaspoon salt
1½ cups mashed banana
¼ cup maple syrup
1 tablespoon vanilla extract
1 cup walnuts, chopped
Directions:
Preheat your oven to 350 degrees F.
Separately, whisk together the dry ingredients in one bowl and the wet ingredients in another bowl.
Beat the two mixtures together until smooth.
Fold in walnuts and give it a gentle stir.
Line a muffin tray with muffin cups and evenly divide the muffin batter among the cups.
Bake for 18 minutes and serve.

Cashew Oat Muffins

Total time: 32 minutes
Ingredients
3 cups rolled oats
¾ cup raw cashews
¼ cup maple syrup
¼ cup sugar
1 teaspoon vanilla extract
½ teaspoon salt
1½ teaspoon baking soda
2 cups water
Directions:
Preheat your oven to 375 degrees F.
Separately, whisk together the dry ingredients in one bowl and the wet ingredients in another bowl.
Beat the two mixtures together until smooth.
Fold in cashews and give it a gentle stir.
Line a muffin tray with muffin cups and evenly divide the muffin batter among the cups.
Bake for 22 minutes and serve.

Banana Cinnamon Muffins

Total time: 32 minutes
Ingredients
3 very ripe bananas, mashed
½ cup vanilla almond milk
1 cup sugar
2 cups flour
1 teaspoon baking soda
½ teaspoon cinnamon
¼ teaspoon salt
Directions:
Preheat your oven to 350 degrees F.
Separately, whisk together the dry ingredients in one bowl and the wet ingredients in another bowl.
Beat the two mixtures together until smooth.
Line a muffin tray with muffin cups and evenly divide the muffin batter among the cups.
Bake for 22 minutes and serve.

Applesauce Muffins

Total time: 35 minutes
Ingredients
2 cups wheat flour
1 tbsp baking powder
1 teaspoon baking soda
½ teaspoon salt
1 teaspoon cinnamon
½ teaspoon ground allspice
½ cup brown sugar
15 ounces apple sauce
½ cup almond milk
1 teaspoon vanilla
1 teaspoon apple cider vinegar
½ cup raisins
½ cup apple, diced
Directions:
Preheat your oven to 350 degrees F.
Separately, whisk together the dry ingredients in one bowl and wet ingredients in another bowl.
Beat the two mixture together until smooth.
Fold in apples and raisins, give it a gentle stir.
Line a muffin tray with muffin cups and evenly divide the muffin batter among the cups.
Bake for nearly 25 minutes and serve.

Chapter 10: Sauces & Dressings Recipes

Cashew Yogurt

Total time: 12 hours 5 minutes
Ingredients
3 probiotic supplements
2 2/3 cups cashews, unsalted , soaked in warm water for 15 minutes
1/4 teaspoon sea salt
4 tablespoon lemon juice
1 1/2 cup water
Directions:
Drain the cashews, add them into the food processor, then add remaining ingredients, except for probiotic supplements, and pulse for 2 minutes until smooth.
Tip the mixture in a bowl, add probiotic supplements, stir until mixed, then cover the bowl with a cheesecloth and let it stand for 12 hours in a dark and cool room.
Serve straight away.

Nacho Cheese Sauce

Total time: 20 minutes
Ingredients
2 cups cashews, unsalted , soaked in warm water for 15 minutes
2 teaspoons salt
1/2 cup nutritional yeast
1 teaspoon garlic powder
1/2 teaspoon smoked paprika
1/2 teaspoon red chili powder
1 teaspoon onion powder
2 teaspoons Sriracha
3 tablespoons lemon juice
4 cups water, divided
Directions:
Drain the cashews, transfer them to a food processor, then add remaining ingredients, reserving 3 cups water, and , and pulse for 3 minutes until smooth.
Tip the mixture in a saucepan, place it over medium heat and cook for 3 to 5 minutes until the sauce has thickened and bubbling, whisking constantly.
When done, taste the sauce to adjust seasoning and then serve.

Spicy Red Wine Tomato Sauce

Total time: 1 hour 5 minutes
Ingredients
28 ounces puree of whole tomatoes, peeled
4 cloves of garlic, peeled
1 tablespoon dried basil
¼ teaspoon ground black pepper
1 tablespoon dried oregano
¼ teaspoon red pepper flakes
1 tablespoon dried sage
1 tablespoon dried thyme
3 teaspoon coconut sugar
1/2 of lemon, juice
1/4 cup red wine
Directions
Take a large saucepan, place it over medium heat, add tomatoes and remaining ingredients, stir and simmer for 1 hour or more until thickened and cooked.
Serve sauce over pasta.

Vodka Cream Sauce

Total time: 10 minutes
Ingredients
1/4 cup cashews, unsalted , soaked in warm water for 15 minutes
24-ounce marinara sauce
2 tablespoons vodka
1/4 cup water
Directions:
Drain the cashews, transfer them in a food processor, pour in water, and blend for 2 minutes until smooth.
Tip the mixture in a pot, stir in pasta sauce and vodka and simmer for 3 minutes over medium heat until done, stirring constantly.
Serve sauce over pasta.

Barbecue Sauce

Total time: 5 minutes
Ingredients
8 ounces tomato sauce
1 teaspoon garlic powder
¼ teaspoon ground black pepper
1/2 teaspoon. sea salt
2 Tablespoons Dijon mustard
3 packets stevia
1 teaspoon molasses
1 Tablespoon apple cider vinegar
2 Tablespoons tamari
1 teaspoon liquid aminos
Directions:
Take a medium bowl, place all the ingredients in it, and stir until combined.
Serve straight away

Bolognese Sauce

Total time: 55 minutes

Ingredients

½ of small green bell pepper, chopped
1 stalk of celery, chopped
1 small carrot, chopped
1 medium white onion, peeled, chopped
2 teaspoons minced garlic
1/2 teaspoon crushed red pepper flakes
3 tablespoons olive oil
8-ounce tempeh, crumbled
8 ounces white mushrooms, chopped
1/2 cup dried red lentils
28-ounce crushed tomatoes
28-ounce whole tomatoes, chopped
1 teaspoon dried oregano
1/2 teaspoon fennel seed
1/2 teaspoon ground black pepper
1/2 teaspoon salt
1 teaspoon dried basil
1/4 cup chopped parsley
1 bay leaf
6-ounce tomato paste
1 cup dry red wine

Directions:

Take a Dutch oven, place it over medium heat, add oil, and when hot, add the first six ingredients, stir and cook for 5 minutes until sauté.

Then switch heat to medium-high level, add two ingredients after olive oil, stir and cook for 3 minutes.

Switch heat to medium-low level, stir in tomato paste, and continue cooking for 2 minutes.

Add remaining ingredients except for lentils, stir and bring the mixture to boil.

Switch heat to the low level, simmer sauce for 10 minutes, covering the pan partially, then add lentils and continue cooking for 20 minutes until tender.

Serve sauce with cooked pasta.

Cilantro and Parsley Hot Sauce

Total time: 5 minutes

Ingredients

2 cups of parsley and cilantro leaves with stems
4 Thai bird chilies, destemmed, deseeded, torn
2 teaspoons minced garlic
1 teaspoon salt
1/4 teaspoon coriander seed, ground
1/4 teaspoon ground black pepper
1/2 teaspoon cumin seeds, ground
3 green cardamom pods, toasted, ground
1/2 cup olive oil

Directions:

Take a spice blender or a food processor, place all the ingredients in it, and process for 5 minutes until the smooth paste comes together.

Serve straight away.

Sweet Mustard Salad Dressing

Total time: 5 minutes
Ingredients
2 tbsp maple syrup
2 tbsp spicy brown mustard
2 tsp rice vinegar
1 cup roasted vidalia onion, pureed* (optional)
Directions:
*Vidalia Onion Option: Gently roast a large vidalia onion and then add it, along with a trip batch of this recipe, to a blender. Sweet onion flavor!

Alfredo Sauce

Total time: 5 minutes
Ingredients
1 cup cashews, unsalted, soaked in warm water for 15 minutes
1 teaspoon minced garlic
1/4 teaspoon ground black pepper
1/3 teaspoon salt
1/4 cup nutritional yeast
2 tablespoons tamari
2 tablespoons olive oil
4 tablespoons water
Directions:
Drain the cashews, transfer them into a food processor, add remaining ingredients in it, and pulse for 3 minutes until thick sauce comes together.
Serve straight away.

Garden Pesto

Total time: 5 minutes
Ingredients
1/4 cup pistachios, shelled
3/4 cup parsley leaves
1 cup cilantro leaves
½ teaspoon minced garlic
1/4 cup mint leaves
1 cup basil leaves
¼ teaspoon ground black pepper
1/3 teaspoon salt
1/2 cup olive oil
1 1/2 teaspoons miso
2 teaspoons lemon juice
Directions:
Place all the ingredients in the order in a food processor or blender and then pulse for 3 to 5 minutes at high speed until smooth.
Tip the pesto in a bowl and then serve.

Hot Sauce

Total time: 25 minutes
Ingredients
4 Serrano peppers, destemmed
1/2 of medium white onion, chopped
1 medium carrot, chopped
10 habanero chilies, destemmed
6 cloves of garlic, unpeeled
2 teaspoons sea salt
1 cup apple cider vinegar
1/2 teaspoon brown rice syrup
1 cup of water
Directions:
Take a skillet pan, place it medium heat, add garlic, and cook for 15 minutes until roasted, frequently turning garlic, set aside to cool.
Meanwhile, take a saucepan, place it over medium-low heat, add remaining ingredients in it, except for salt and syrup, stir and cook for 12 minutes until vegetables are tender.
When the garlic has roasted and cooled, peel them and add them to a food processor.
Then add cooked saucepan along with remaining ingredients, and pulse for 3 minutes until smooth.
Let sauce cool and then serve straight away

Hot Sauce

Total time: 5 minutes
Ingredients
4 cloves of garlic, peeled
15 Hot peppers, de-stemmed, chopped
1/2 teaspoon. coriander
1/2 teaspoon. sea salt
1/2 teaspoon. red chili powder
1/2 of lime, zested
1/4 teaspoon. cumin
1/2 lime, juiced
1 cup apple cider vinegar
Directions:
Place all the ingredients in the order in a food processor or blender and then pulse for 3 to 5 minutes at high speed until smooth.
Tip the sauce in a bowl and then serve.

Thai Peanut Sauce

Total time: 20 minutes
Ingredients
2 tablespoons ground peanut, and more for topping
2 tablespoons Thai red curry paste
½ teaspoon salt
1 tablespoon sugar
1/2 cup creamy peanut butter
2 tablespoons apple cider vinegar
3/4 cup coconut milk, unsweetened
Directions:
Take a saucepan, place it over low heat, add all the ingredients, whisk well until combined, and then bring the sauce to simmer.
Then remove the pan from heat, top with ground peanuts, and serve.

Garlic Alfredo Sauce

Total time: 15 minutes
 Ingredients
1 1/2 cups cashews, unsalted , soaked in warm water for 15 minutes
6 cloves of garlic, peeled, minced
1/2 medium sweet onion, peeled, chopped
1 teaspoon salt
1/4 cup nutritional yeast
1 tablespoon lemon juice
2 tablespoons olive oil
2 cups almond milk, unsweetened
12 ounces fettuccine pasta, cooked, for serving
Directions:
Take a small saucepan, place it over medium heat, add oil and when hot, add onion and garlic, and cook for 5 minutes until sauté.
Meanwhile, drain the cashews, transfer them into a food processor, add remaining ingredients including onion mixture, except for pasta, and pulse for 3 minutes until very smooth.
Pour the prepared sauce over pasta, toss until coated and serve.

Buffalo Chicken Dip

Total time: 20 minutes
Ingredients
2 cups cashews
2 teaspoons garlic powder
1 1/2 teaspoons salt
2 teaspoons onion powder
3 tablespoons lemon juice
1 cup buffalo sauce
1 cup of water
14-ounce artichoke hearts, packed in water, drained
Directions:
Switch on the oven, then set it to 375 degrees F and let it preheat.
Meanwhile, pour 3 cups of boiling water in a bowl, add cashews and let soak for 5 minutes.
Then drain the cashew, transfer them into the blender, pour in water, add lemon juice and all the seasoning and blend until smooth.
Add artichokes and buffalo sauce, process until chunky mixture comes together, and then transfer the dip to an ovenproof dish.
Bake for 20 minutes and then serve.

Barbecue Tahini Sauce

Total time: 5 minutes
 Ingredients
6 tablespoons tahini
3/4 teaspoon garlic powder
1/8 teaspoon red chili powder
2 teaspoons maple syrup
1/4 teaspoon salt
3 teaspoons molasses
3 teaspoons apple cider vinegar
1/4 teaspoon liquid smoke
10 teaspoons tomato paste
1/2 cup water
Directions:
Place all the ingredients in the order in a food processor or blender and then pulse for 3 to 5 minutes at high speed until smooth.
Tip the sauce in a bowl and then serve.

Vegan Ranch Dressing

Total time: 5 minutes
 Ingredients
1/4 teaspoon. ground black pepper
2 teaspoon. chopped parsley
1/2 teaspoon. garlic powder
1 tablespoon chopped dill
1/2 teaspoon. onion powder
1 cup vegan mayonnaise
1/2 cup soy milk, unsweetened
Directions:
Take a medium bowl, add all the ingredients in it and then whisk until combined.
Serve straight away

Sweet Mustard Salad Dressing

Total time: 10 minutes
Ingredients
2 tbsp maple syrup
2 tbsp spicy brown mustard
2 tsp rice vinegar
1 cup roasted vidalia onion, pureed* (optional)
Directions:
*Vidalia Onion Option: Gently roast a large vidalia onion and then add it, along with a trip batch of this recipe, to a blender. Sweet onion flavor!

Spiced Peach Compote

Total time: 17 minutes
Ingredients
1 ½ cups fresh or frozen peaches, peeled and pitted, chopped small
2 tbsp water
½ tsp pumpkin pie spice blend
¼ tsp vanilla
Directions:
1 tbsp cornstarch mixed into 2 tbsp water (cornstarch slurry)
 In a small saucepan over medium heat, add first four ingredients and mix together. Allow to come to a simmer and cook for 7 minutes.
Mash lightly and add the cornstarch slurry.
Bring back to a simmer and then remove from heat.
Allow to cool slightly and thicken before serving.

Tzatziki Sauce

Total time: 40 minutes
Ingredients.
 ¼ cup raw cashews, soaked in boiling water for 15 min
¼ cup white potatoes, peeled, boiled, and diced small
1 tsp dry dill (fresh if available)
½ tsp powdered garlic (or 1 clove finely minced)
½ med. cucumber, unpeeled (about ⅓ cup grated)
½ cup plant milk, unsweetened OR liquid from cucumber
1 lemon, juice & zest
½ tsp apple cider vinegar
Directions:
Finely grate the cucumber into a thin tea towel, then squeeze the liquid out into a bowl until mostly dry. Save the liquid.
Into a wide mouth quart jar, add: juice & zest of one lemon, vinegar, dill, garlic, soaked cashews, potatoes and almond milk or equivalent cucumber liquid.
Using an immersion blender, blend until creamy.
Add cucumber and blend some more. Add a bit more almond milk or cucumber liquid to thin if necessary.
Allow to rest in the refrigerator for 30 minutes before using.

BBQ Sauce

Total time: 10 minutes
Ingredients
½ cup diced bell pepper, sauteed
½ cup diced sweet onion, sauteed
1 cup ketchup OR 3 tbsp tomato paste and ½ cup water
3 tbsp brown mustard
1/4 cup maple syrup
1/2 cup water
1 tsp liquid smoke
Directions:
Process all of the ingredients in a blender, store in an airtight container in the refrigerator.

Creamy Corn Sauce

Total time: 15 minutes
Ingredients
1 tablespoon vegan butter
2 garlic cloves, minced
1 tablespoon all-purpose flour
1 ¾ cups full-fat coconut milk
2 tablespoons nutritional yeast
½ teaspoon salt
½ teaspoon black pepper
3 cups corn kernels
Directions:
Place a medium-sized skillet over medium heat and add vegan butter.
Stir in garlic and sauté for 30 seconds, then stir in flour.
Whisk well and cook for another 30 seconds, then stir in salt, coconut milk, yeast, and black pepper.
Stir for 1 minute then add corn kernels.
Cook for 2 minutes then serve.

Cranberry Sauce

Total time: 25 minutes
Ingredients
12 oz fresh cranberries
1 cup of sugar
1 cup of water
1 lemon, zested
Directions:
Dump all the ingredients into a medium-sized saucepan.
Let it simmer for 15 minutes until the sauce thickens.
Serve.

Soy Ranch Dressing

Total time: 10 minutes
Ingredients
1 cup mayonnaise
1½ teaspoon garlic finely powdered
½ teaspoon onion finely powdered
¼ teaspoon pepper powder
2 teaspoons parsley, chopped
1 tablespoon dill, chopped
½ cup soy milk
Directions:
Dump all the ranch dressing ingredients into a blender jug.
Blend the dressing mixture for 1 minute.
Serve.

Chili Marinara Sauce

Total time: 60 minutes
Ingredients
- 4 tbsp olive oil
- 1 small white onion, chopped
- 5 garlic cloves, minced
- 10 cups fresh tomatoes, crushed
- 4 tbsp tomato paste
- Salt and black pepper to taste
- ½ cup red wine
- ½ cup water
- 2 tsp dried basil
- 2 tsp dried oregano
- 2 tbsp dried parsley
- 2 tbsp Italian seasoning
- 1 tsp pure maple syrup
- 1 tsp red chili powder

Directions:
Heat the olive oil in a pot over medium heat and sauté the onion to make it soft, 3 minutes. Mix in the garlic and cook until fragrant, 30 seconds.
Pour in the remaining ingredients, stir, and close the lid.
Bring the ingredients to a boil, then reduce the heat to low, and simmer until the tomatoes are very soft, 30 to 40 minutes.
Open the lid and using an immersion blender, puree the ingredients until smooth.
Spoon the sauce into jars.
Use for stews, pasta, and rice dishes.

Onion Gravy with Red Onion

Total time: 15 minutes
Ingredients
2 tbsp plant butter
- 1 shallot, finely chopped
- 1 tsp whole-wheat flour
- 1 tbsp red wine vinegar
- 2 cups red wine
- 1 cup thinly sliced red onion
- 1 cup vegetable stock
- 1 tsp dried oregano
- 1 tbsp Dijon mustard
- 1 tbsp cornstarch
- Salt to taste

Directions:
Melt half of the butter in a medium pot and sauté the shallots until softened, 2 minutes. Mix in the flour until breadcrumb-like mixture forms.
Mix in the red wine vinegar until thick paste forms and then, stir in the red wine.
Add the vegetable stock, oregano, and Dijon mustard. Combine well and allow simmering for 3 to 5 minutes.
Whisk in the cornstarch and cook until the sauce thickens, 1 to 2 minutes.
Season with a little salt, spoon into serving cups and use over or with grilled vegetables, tofu, seitan, etc.

Velote Sauce

Total time: 10 minutes
Ingredients
- 2 tbsp unsalted plant butter
- 2 tbsp whole-wheat flour
- 1 cup vegetable broth, warmed
- 3 tbsp cashew cream
- ½ lemon, juiced
- Salt and black pepper to taste

Directions:
1. Melt the plant butter in a medium pot over medium heat and whisk in the flour; cook until golden, 1 minute.
2. Mix in the vegetable broth until smooth and cook until the sauce is slightly syrupy, 2 to 3 minutes. Turn the heat off.
3. Vigorously whisk in the cashew cream, lemon juice, salt, and black pepper.
4. Spoon the sauce into serving cups and use over grilled vegetables and plant-protein options.

Tangy Pea Butter Sauce

Total time: 20 minutes
Ingredients
- 1 cup unsalted plant butter
- 1 garlic clove, minced
- ¼ cup chopped fresh cilantro
- 1 cup fresh garden peas
- ½ cup vegetable broth
- 2 limes, juiced
- Salt and black pepper to taste

Directions:
Melt the plant butter in a large pot and sauté the garlic until fragrant, 30 seconds.
Mix in the remaining ingredients, cover the pot, and simmer until the peas are very soft, 10 to 15 minutes.
Open the lid and transfer the food to a blender. Process until smooth.
Pour the sauce into serving cups and use immediately with grilled vegetables, tofu, tempeh, etc.

Alfredo Sauce

Total time: 15 minutes
Ingredients
- ½ cup vegetable broth
- 4 garlic cloves, minced
- 4 leaves fresh basil, chopped
- ¼ cup freshly chopped parsley
- 4 tbsp plant butter
- 2 cups coconut cream
- 8 oz cashew cheese, softened
- 1 cup grated plant-based Parmesan cheese

Directions:
Combine the vegetable broth, garlic, basil, and parsley in a medium pot and simmer over low heat for 10 minutes.
Stir in the plant butter, coconut cream, cashew cheese, and plant-based Parmesan cheese until the cheeses melt.
Use the sauce immediately for Alfredo pasta dishes.

Garlic Alfredo Sauce

Total time: 22 minutes
Ingredients
1 medium white onion, diced
2 cups vegetable broth
½ teaspoon salt
½ teaspoon ground black pepper
4 garlic cloves, minced
½ cup raw cashews
2 tablespoons lemon juice
4 tablespoons nutritional yeast
Directions:
Cook onion with 1 cup broth in a large pan for 8 minutes over medium heat.
Stir in garlic and cook for another 4 minutes until it is creamy.
Puree this veggie mixture in a blender jug.
Now add remaining broth, black pepper, salt, cashews, nutritional yeast, and lemon juice.
Blend well until smooth.
Enjoy.

Molasses Tahini Sauce

Total time: 10 minutes
Ingredients
6 tablespoons tahini
10 teaspoons tomato paste
2 teaspoons maple syrup
¾ teaspoon garlic powder
3 teaspoons apple cider vinegar
3 teaspoons molasses
¼ teaspoon liquid smoke
Sea salt, to taste
1/8 teaspoon chili powder
½ cup water
Directions:
Dump all the tahini sauce ingredients into a blender jug.
Blend the tahini mixture for 2 minutes.
Serve.

Teriyaki Sauce

Total time: 10 minutes
Ingredients!
1 tbsp soy sauce or tamari or coconut aminos
1 tsp ginger, powdered
1 tsp garlic, powdered
1 tbsp maple syrup
1 tbsp tahini
¼ cup water
3 tbsp sesame seeds
Directions:
In a small saucepan, whisk together the first 5 ingredients.
Over medium heat, bring the mixture to a simmer and allow to cook, covered, for 5 minutes.
Immediately remove from the heat and allow to cool slightly.
In a dry skillet over medium heat, lightly toast 3 tbsp sesame seeds.
Add sesame seeds to the sauce right before serving.

White 'Cream' Sauce

Total time: 10 minutes
Ingredients
1 ½ cup plant milk, unsweetened
⅓ cup cooked chickpeas
½ cup aquafaba or water
¼ cup raw cashews, soaked in boiling water for 10 min, then rinsed and drained OR
1 cup boiled yukon gold potatoes, cubed
1 tbsp lemon juice
1 tbsp Dijon mustard
1 1/2 tbsp cornstarch dissolved in 3 tbsp water
1 tbsp miso paste
1 tsp thyme, dried
1/2 tsp freshly ground black pepper
1 tsp garlic powder
1 tsp onion powder
Directions:
Blend all ingredients together until smooth.

Blueberry Sauce

Total time: 13 minutes
Ingredients
3/4 cup blueberries
¼ tsp cinnamon
Pinch of powdered cloves
½ tsp vanilla
2 tbsp water
Directions:
In a small saucepan, bring all the ingredients to a simmer and mash the berries slightly.
Allow to simmer for 3 minutes, then turn off the heat.
Allow berries to rest for 5 minutes.

Cranberry Mandarin Sauce

Total time: 17 minutes
Ingredients
1 cup cranberries
1 cup raisins
1 ½ cup water, divided
2 peeled mandarin oranges, diced
½ tsp cinnamon
Directions:
1/16 tsp (a pinch!) each of ground mace, allspice, cloves
In a small saucepan, bring ¾ cup of water to a boil, add the fruit, juice, and spices, and simmer on low for 7 minutes.
When raisins are soft and cranberries are splitting, add everything to a blender, add the remaining water, and blend until smooth.
Should be a smooth, spreadable viscosity.

CPSIA information can be obtained
at www.ICGtesting.com
Printed in the USA
BVHW052002131021
618835BV00004B/296